MEASURING PATIENT SAFETY

EDITED BY

Robin Newhouse, RN, PhD
The Johns Hopkins Hospital
The Johns Hopkins University School of Nursing

Stephanie Poe, RN, MScN
The Johns Hopkins Hospital

JONES AND BARTLETT PUBLISHERS
Sudbury, Massachusetts
BOSTON   TORONTO   LONDON   SINGAPORE

World Headquarters
Jones and Bartlett Publishers
40 Tall Pine Drive
Sudbury, MA 01776
978-443-5000
info@jbpub.com
www.jbpub.com

Jones and Bartlett Publishers
Canada
2406 Nikanna Road
Mississauga, ON L5C 2W6
CANADA

Jones and Bartlett Publishers
International
Barb House, Barb Mews
London W6 7PA
UK

Library of Congress Cataloging-in-Publication Data

Measuring patient safety / editors, Robin P. Newhouse & Stephanie S. Poe.
    p. ; cm.
 Includes bibliographical references.
 ISBN 0-7637-2841-1
 1. Hospitals—Safety measures. 2. Patients—Safety measures. 3. Nursing.
 [DNLM: 1. Hospitals. 2. Medical Errors—prevention & control--Nurses' Instruction. 3. Outcome Assessment (Health Care)—Nurses' Instruction. 4. Patient Satisfaction—Nurses' Instruction. 5. Risk Assessment—Nurses' Instruction. 6. Safety Management—Nurses' Instruction. 7. Self-Evaluation Programs—Nurses' Instruction. WX 153 M484 2005] I. Newhouse, Robin Purdy. II. Poe, Stephanie S.
 RA969.9.M43 2005
 363.15'7--dc22

2004012546

Production Credits
Acquisitions Editor: Kevin Sullivan
Production Manager: Amy Rose
Associate Production Editor: Karen C. Ferreira
Editorial Assistant: Amy Sibley
Marketing Manager: Ed McKenna
Associate Marketing Manager: Emily Ekle
Manufacturing and Inventory Coordinator: Amy Bacus
Composition and Design: Paw Print Media
Cover Design: Anne Spencer
Printing and Binding: Courier Stoughton
Cover Printing: Courier Stoughton
Cover Images: Top photo courtesy of MIEMSS. Other photos © Photodisc.

Printed in the United States of America
08 07 06 05 04   10 9 8 7 6 5 4 3 2 1

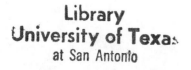

To nurses: working together to improve safety for patients.
My precious family—Frank, Kirsten, A.J., Tristan, Kristie, and
Laszlo—for your continuous love and support.

—Robin

My husband and best friend André; our children Danielle,
Michael, and Nicholas; and my parents Hilda and Pat for your
never-ending faith in me.

—Stephanie

Contributors and Affiliations

Sean Berenholtz, MD, MHS
The Johns Hopkins University School of Medicine

Donna Brannan, RN, MSN
The Johns Hopkins Hospital

Patricia B. Dawson, RN, MSN
The Johns Hopkins Hospital

Todd Dorman, MD
The Johns Hopkins University School of Medicine

Gary Dunn, RN, MAS, MSN
The Johns Hopkins Hospital

Geetha Jayaram, MD, MBA
The Johns Hopkins University School of Medicine

Bernard Vincent Keenan, RN, BC, MSN
The Johns Hopkins Hospital,
The Johns Hopkins University School of Nursing

Dina Krenzischek, MAS, RN, CPAN
The Johns Hopkins Hospital

Terry Nelson, RN, MSN
The Johns Hopkins Hospital

Robin Newhouse, RN, PhD
The Johns Hopkins Hospital,
The Johns Hopkins University School of Nursing

MiKeala Olsen, RN, MS, OCN
The Johns Hopkins Hospital

Stephanie Poe, RN, MScN
The Johns Hopkins Hospital

Judith Rohde, RN, MS
The Johns Hopkins Hospital

Mandy Schwarz, RN, NCIIIe
The Johns Hopkins Hospital

Sharon Strobel, RN, MS
The Johns Hopkins Hospital

Karin Taylor, APRN, PMH
The Johns Hopkins Hospital

Pedro Mendez-Tellez, MD
The Johns Hopkins University School of Medicine

Rhonda Wyskiel, RN, BSN
The Johns Hopkins Hospital

Table of Contents

Introduction   **xi**

1   Patient Safety as a Measure of Healthcare Quality   1

     What Is Quality? 2

     How Large Is the Patient Safety Problem? 3

     How Do We Improve Quality of Care? 4

          Evidence-Based Practice 4

          Professional Education and Development 5

          Regular Assessments of Clinical Performance
             and Public Accountability 6

          Patient-Centered Care 6

          Total Quality Management 6

          Performance Improvement through Measurement 6

          Patient Safety as a Measure of Healthcare Quality 7

     Why Should Nurses Measure Safety Outcomes? 9

     Conclusion 10

     References 10

2   Using Performance Improvement to Support Patient Safety   13

     Codification of Safety Principles 14

     Alignment of Safety and Performance Improvement 15

     Enabling Staff Participation 17

     Priority Performance Improvement Topics 17

          Sentinel Events and Patient Safety Goals 18

          Hospital-Acquired Infection 18

          Medication Safety 20

          Nurse-Sensitive Safety Measures 21

     Communicating Successes 22

     Recommendations for Nurse Leaders 23

Conclusion 23

References 23

3 Moving Forward: Planning a Safety Project   27

Assumptions and Realities 28

A Comprehensive Patient Safety Program 28

Step 1: Safety Climate Survey *29*

Step 2: The Science of Safety Education *30*

Step 3: Staff Survey *31*

Step 4: Taking an In-Depth Look *31*

Step 5: Plan and Implement Improvements *33*

Steps 6 and 7: Document the Results and Share the Stories *35*

Step 8: Resurvey Staff *35*

Role of the Nurse in Planning a Safety Project 35

Making the Vision a Reality *36*

Fostering Collaboration and Patient-Centered Health Care *36*

Competency in Data Management and Analytical Skills *37*

Conclusion 37

References 38

4 Rapid Cycle Safety Improvement   39

Current Quality Improvement Methods 40

The Model for Improvement 40

Reflection: The Critical Questions *41*

Action *43*

Case Study 47

What Were We Trying to Accomplish? *47*

How Would We Know That Change Was an Improvement? *47*

*What Changes Could We Make That Would Result
    in Improvement?* *48*

PDSA *48*

Conclusion 49

References 49

5 The Metrics of Measuring Patient Safety   51

Selecting a Patient Safety Measure 52

Identifying the Problem to Be Measured *53*

Team Decisions *54*

Locating Examples of Measures *60*

Safety Measures of Structure, Process, and Outcome 60
 Should You Measure Structure, Process, or Outcome? *61*
Conclusion 63
References 64

6 Dissemination of Findings   67

Internal and External Dissemination 68
 Internal Dissemination *69*
 External Dissemination *69*
Comparative Study between Bedside and
 Laboratory Hemoglobin Testing 77
Conclusion 78
References 78

7 Safer Care for Patients on Mechanical Ventilation   79

What Was Our Goal? 80
How Would We Know When We Reached Our Goal? 81
What Changes Could We Make
 That Would Result in an Improvement? 82
 Plan *84*
 Do *84*
 Study *84*
 Act *84*
Conclusion 85
References 85

8 Medication Reconciliation in the ICU   89

Background 89
Plan 90
Do 90
Study 90
Act 91
Lessons Learned 92
Conclusion 94

9 Chemotherapy Safety   95

Background 96
Plan 96
Do 97

Study 103

Act 103

Conclusion 105

Reference 105

**10   Preventing Patient Aggression:
Assessment and Reporting as First Steps   107**

Background 108

Results 108

Plan 110

Do 113

Study 115

Act 118

Conclusion 119

References 119

11   Resources for Conducting a Safety Project   121

City, State, and Federal Government Resources 123

Drug Information 124

Medical and Nursing Directories, Indexes, and Clinical Resources 124

Professional Organizations and Associations 127

Research 133

Miscellaneous Safety Sites 134

Search Engines 136

**Appendix: The Johns Hopkins Hospital
Performance Improvement Workbook   137**

Index   145

Introduction

The prevalence of medical errors, along with widespread recognition of the need for rapid changes in the healthcare system to reduce the incidence of preventable adverse medical events, has grown exponentially since the publication of two landmark Institute of Medicine (IOM) reports: *To Err Is Human: Building a Better Health Care System* (1999) and *Crossing the Quality Chasm: A New Health System for the 21st Century* (2001). The urgency of providing safe environments for patients has been made evident through evolving research, public response, and regulatory changes. The issue of patient safety has been far more intimate for nurses, who work at the bedside and are at the forefront of health care delivery.

Nurses' professional commitment is built on respect for human dignity and dedication to protect and preserve life. In protecting patients from harm through safety initiatives, nurses can use their expertise and organizational knowledge to directly reduce the risk of injury to patients. The urgency of patient safety requires nurses to take a leadership role in measuring and improving the structures, processes, and patient outcomes in the clinical setting.

Purpose of the Book

This book is intended to provide nurses with the basic knowledge and skills needed to participate in and lead multidisciplinary safety initiatives. Nurses who are clinical leaders, managers, and educators who are committed to making our healthcare system safer will explore the concepts and processes associated with measuring and improving patient safety. The chapters will include a background on safety, examples of successful safety projects and lessons learned, measures of safety, practical tips on planning a safety project, resources for safety projects, recommendations on communicating results of projects, and using the Plan-Do-Study-Act (PDSA) framework to create a safety project. This book will help prepare nurses to assess and measure phenomena related to patient safety. These skills are necessary because of the acute importance of healthcare safety, and the integral part that nurses play in the multidisciplinary team. Nurses are often the drivers of safety initiatives, and need to be confident in their skills and knowledge to measure and improve processes that impact patient safety.

Overview of Chapters

Chapter 1, "Patient Safety as a Measure of Healthcare Quality," provides the context for viewing safety as an urgent priority. The concept of quality of care will be discussed, as it relates specifically to patient safety, and the scope of the patient safety problem will be quantified. A general discussion of approaches to improving quality will include evidence-based practice (EBP) and evidence-based clinical practice guidelines, professional education and development, assessment and accountability, patient-centered care, and total quality management. Patient safety will be identified as a measure of healthcare quality, and the underpinnings of error reduction will be introduced. The chapter will close with a discussion of the importance of nurses in measuring safety outcomes. Recommendations will be proposed for nurse leaders to successfully promote measuring patient safety, with the overall goal of quality and safety in patient care. The objectives of Chapter 1 are to:

- Define quality as a multidimensional construct
- Discuss the scope of the patient safety problem
- Discuss approaches to improving quality of care
- Identify patient safety as a measure of healthcare quality
- Discuss why nurses should measure safety outcomes

Chapter 2, "Using Performance Improvement to Support Patient Safety," will provide an understanding of how organizational performance improvement (PI) structures and processes can be used to support patient safety initiatives. Content will include how organizations have integrated safety principles into PI activities. Organizations have aligned PI structures and processes based on internal and external patient safety priorities, enabling staff nurses to actively participate in interdisciplinary PI teams that design and implement patient safety projects. Organizational development of safety initiatives and the importance of communication within the organization, so that important lessons learned will be disseminated, will be discussed. The chapter will close with recommendations for nurse leaders to successfully integrate patient safety into PI programs, with the overall goal of quality and safety in patient care. Chapter 2's objectives are to:

- Discuss how the organization has codified safety principles
- Link PI structures and processes with internally and externally driven patient safety priorities

- Describe how PI enables staff nurses to actively participate in interdisciplinary patient safety projects
- Explore methods to develop and communicate measures of success

Chapter 3, "Moving Forward: Planning a Safety Project," will concentrate on how to move a safety project forward through planning and a systematic approach. Nurse leaders will gain practical insight into the process, and build knowledge needed to lead a safety project. A structured approach for planning and implementing a safety project will be detailed. The role of the nurse as a member of the multidisciplinary safety team will be included, with a discussion of successful strategies for nurses' personal growth. Chapter 3's objectives are to:

- Describe the steps in planning a safety project
- Discuss the role of the nurse as a member of the multidisciplinary safety team

Chapter 4, "Rapid Cycle Safety Improvement," introduces the concept of rapid cycle methodologies for PI. This chapter is a toolbox for rapid cycle change. Current quality improvement methods will be discussed, and the PDSA Model for Improvement will be described. Critical questions before embarking on change will be posed. This chapter is the "how to" for PDSA cycles for testing change. The chapter will close with an example of how the Model for Improvement was used to enhance medication safety in a medical intensive care unit. The objectives of Chapter 4 are to:

- Describe current quality improvement methods
- Describe the Model for Improvement
- Identify critical questions to answer before embarking on change
- Describe how to use PDSA cycles for testing changes
- Describe how the Model for Improvement was used to enhance medication safety in a medical intensive care unit

Chapter 5, "The Metrics of Measuring Patient Safety," focuses on appropriate measures to use to capture safety improvements. Strong measurement allows teams to articulate, both within the organization and externally to professional or policy audiences, the impact of improvements to their unit. The process of selecting a patient safety measure will be described. Structure, process, and the outcome of patient safety measures will be introduced with examples and tools that can be used by safety teams. Skill in measurement and interpretation of outcomes are essential for nurse leaders involved in safety initiatives, and they will serve them well, building their professional credibility and value to the team. The objectives of Chapter 5 are to:

- Describe the process for selecting a patient safety measure
- Identify patient safety measures of structure, process, and outcome

Chapter 6, "Dissemination of Findings," focuses on how to disseminate the findings of safety projects, both internally within the organization and externally through professional networks. The importance of dissemination of findings and lessons from safety projects is stressed. Practical examples, successful strategies, and guidelines for poster or oral presentations and publication are included. Through dissemination, nurses can develop a leadership position in measuring patient safety. The objectives of Chapter 6 are to:

■ Describe the internal and external organizational dissemination processes

■ Identify opportunities for presentation of safety project outcomes

■ Discuss successful presentation strategies

Chapters 7, 8, 9, and 10 provide exemplars of patient safety projects. These exemplars include the team's approach to the problem, the process for improvement, and the outcomes using the PDSA cycle. These four projects include a variety of focuses: evidence-based practice for ventilated patients, continuity of care in transfer orders, processes of chemotherapy administration, and identification of factors to assess and reduce episodes of patient violence.

■ Chapter 7, "Safer Care for Patients on Mechanical Ventilation," describes the development of an integrated approach to improving safety in an intensive care unit (ICU), coupled with the concepts of care bundles, independent redundancy, and reducing complexity to enhance provider compliance with the use of evidence-based therapies.

■ Chapter 8, "Medication Reconciliation in the ICU," discusses a continuum of care project that implemented medication reconciliation in the ICU.

■ Chapter 9, "Chemotherapy Safety," demonstrates a project to reduce chemotherapy errors in an era when novel classes of chemotherapy and biotherapy agents, as well as new combinations of treatment modalities, are emerging.

■ Chapter 10, "Preventing Patient Aggression," describes a performance improvement initiative to enable nurses to identify patients who have a greater propensity for aggression so that they can implement appropriate interventions before the violence escalates.

Chapter 11, "Resources for Conducting a Safety Project," provides a list of safety-related internal and external resources for safety teams. This list explores networks, publications, organizations, and web sites that will be valuable assets for any safety improvement project. The objective of Chapter 11 is to identify resources available for the conduct of safety projects.

Conclusion

This book content was based on presentations delivered in "Measuring Safety," a two-day seminar conducted three times between October 2002 and November 2003 at the Johns Hopkins Hospital. Attendees were nurses, who went on to successfully conduct safety projects in their clinical areas. On follow-up evaluation, participants endorsed the attendance at this two-day conference as content necessary for any nurse involved in safety initiatives. Seventy-nine percent went on to become actively engaged in safety projects, using the knowledge and skills built through this content. Through publishing this book, it is our hope that you also will benefit from our lessons learned, joining in the effort to create safe healthcare environments for patients.

CHAPTER 1

Patient Safety as a Measure of Healthcare Quality

Todd Dorman, MD, Associate Professor[*][#]
Sean Berenholtz, MD, MHS, Assistant Professor[*]
Pedro Mendez-Tellez, MD, Assistant Professor[*]
Stephanie S. Poe, MScN, RN, Coordinator for Nursing Clinical Quality[◆]
Robin Newhouse, PhD, RN, Nurse Researcher, Assistant Professor[#][◆]

You have noticed that patient safety has been given a lot of press time lately. Hardly a day goes by in which a newspaper article or television news program does not mention a new event related to medical error. As a nurse, you have always been concerned about the safety of your patients. You have noticed a variety of situations that place your patients at risk, but have been hesitant to "rock the boat." You have heard that your hospital has developed a Patient Safety Program, and you wonder what your role will be in this process. "Patient safety" appears to be a popular topic at the moment, but will things ever really change?

Patient safety and improvement of healthcare quality is of paramount importance to nurses. Integral provisions of the Code of Ethics for Nurses (American Nurses Association [ANA], 2001) are the nurse's role in protecting the patient's safety and his or her participation in establishing, maintaining, and improving the healthcare environment to provide quality health care. That nurses, as the most consistent presence at the patient's bedside, play a significant role in initiatives to improve the systems and processes of care is not surprising.

What is unexpected, however, is the public's heightened awareness of the prevalence of medical error and widespread recognition of the need for rapid

[*]Department of Anesthesiology and Critical Care Medicine
 The Johns Hopkins University School of Medicine
[#]The Johns Hopkins School of Nursing
[◆]Department of Nursing, The Johns Hopkins Hospital

changes in the healthcare system to reduce the incidence of preventable adverse medical events. Responsiveness to patient safety issues has grown exponentially since the publication of the two landmark Institute of Medicine (IOM) reports entitled *To Err Is Human: Building a Better Health Care System* (1999) and *Crossing the Quality Chasm: A New Health System for the 21st Century* (2001). A subsequent report, *Keeping Patients Safe: Transforming the Work Environment for Nurses* (2004), takes an additional step in linking nurses directly with safety. "Research is now beginning to document what physicians, patients, other health care providers, and nurses themselves have long known: how well we are cared for by nurses affects our health, and sometimes can be a matter of life or death" (IOM, 2004, p. 2).

Published literature and Internet communication lines are bursting with accounts of federal, state, regulatory, professional, and private sector efforts to refocus performance improvement (PI) activities on developing safer systems and processes of care. The need to measure whether changes implemented as a result of these activities actually succeed in making care safer has become even more important with the growth of public reporting mandates.

The overall aim of this chapter is to provide clinical nurse leaders, educators, and managers with an understanding of the role of patient safety in measuring quality of care. The objectives of this chapter are to:

- Define quality as a multidimensional construct
- Discuss the scope of the patient safety problem
- Discuss approaches to improving quality of care
- Identify patient safety as a measure of healthcare quality
- Discuss why nurses should measure safety outcomes

The chapter will close with recommendations for nurse leaders to successfully promote measuring patient safety, with the overall goal of quality and safety in patient care.

What Is Quality?

Quality is a multidimensional construct (Blumenthal, 1996). The IOM defines healthcare quality as "the degree to which health services for individuals and populations increase the likelihood of desired health outcomes and are consistent with current professional knowledge" (IOM, 2003). This definition suggests a broad approach to measuring healthcare quality in terms of the type of data measured, desired outcomes, and related processes of care. As such, to get a true picture of the quality of care that we provide, we will likely require a measurement system that includes a combination of process (what we do) and outcome (the results of care) measures. In addition, depending on whose perspective (patient, providers, hospital, insurers, regulators) you have, certain aspects or domains of quality may be more important (McGlynn, 1998; McGlynn & Ashe, 1998). For example, providers generally care more about biologic outcomes, such as response to therapy; patients generally care more about symptoms; and payers generally care more about costs. The IOM report, *Crossing the Quality Chasm*, outlines six domains of quality that provide a framework for all quality measures (IOM, 2001). These domains are grounded in the notion that health care should be safe, effective, efficient, patient-centered, timely, and equitable. These aims serve as a framework for considering the domains of quality and for evaluating the impact of quality improvement initiatives.

How Large Is the Patient Safety Problem?

The opportunity that we have to improve the care we provide to our patients is substantial (Chassin & Galvin, 1998; President's Advisory Commission, 1998). The IOM estimates that 44,000–98,000 preventable deaths occur every year in U.S. hospitals (IOM, 1999). Although the epidemiology of preventable deaths has been avidly debated, these estimates have survived the challenges (Leape, 2000). Even if the lower estimate of preventable deaths is used (44,000 per year), this represents more annual deaths in the United States than those caused by diseases like AIDS and breast cancer or from motor vehicle accidents. Stated in other terms, the number of preventable annual deaths is greater than the total number of deaths that would occur if a 747 airplane crashed and killed all its passengers every other day for a year.

As members of healthcare teams practicing in complex systems of care, and as patients and family members who must access the healthcare system, nurses are acutely aware of the unfortunate numbers of adverse events and near misses that occur. They are not as aware, however, that most of these events are preventable and that nurses play a critical role in working with interdisciplinary teams to identify and remedy system flaws that predispose these events to occur. Donald Berwick has repeatedly stated that every system is perfectly designed to deliver the results it gets. Consequently, we all need to focus on improving our systems of care.

It may be easy for you to recall an instance where a flaw in the system has led to a significant medical error. An example of such an instance involved the administration of undiluted esmolol hydrochloride (Brevibloc®) from a syringe that had been prepared by an inexperienced nurse team member. What had begun as a manageable emergency situation progressed to a critical event. After the patient had been stabilized, the team reviewed the event and it was revealed that the nurse had not seen a warning printed on the drug ampule that this drug must be diluted prior to administration. The nurse who provided the esmolol did not label the syringe and the physician who administered the drug did not inquire as to the concentration. Despite a large red tag on the esmolol vial (Figure 1.1) stating that the drug must be diluted, the warning was insufficient to prevent providers from proceeding without dilution. A compounding factor was that two different concentrations of esmolol were routinely available (one dilute, one concentrated). The dilute form was out-of-stock, and the nurse team member had to draw from the concentrated form.

Figure 1.1   Large Visible Labels Do Not Always Prevent Medication Errors

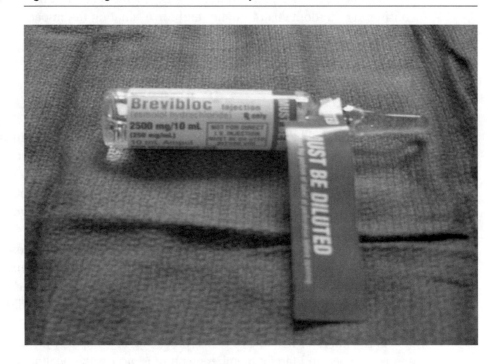

How Do We Improve Quality of Care?

There are multiple approaches to improving quality of care (Grol, 2001). These methods include evidence-based practice (EBP) and evidence-based clinical practice guidelines, professional education and development, assessment and accountability, patient-centered care, and total quality management (Grol, 2001). Table 1.1 presents the underlying assumptions of these approaches.

Evidence-Based Practice

The premise of EBP and evidence-based clinical practice guidelines is that we can improve clinical decision making and patient care by incorporating the best available evidence with patient values and provider preferences (Sackett et al., 1996). Guidelines and protocols have been successful in improving performance with some care processes. For example, sedation and ventilator weaning protocols have been shown to decrease the duration of mechanical ventilation and

Table 1.1   Approaches to Improving Quality of Care

Approach	Assumptions
Evidence-based medicine, clinical practice guidelines, decision aids	Provision of best evidence and convincing information leads to optimal decision making and optimal care.
Professional education and development, self-regulation, recertification	Bottom-up learning based on experiences in practice and individual learning needs leads to performance change.
Assessment and accountability feedback, accreditation, public reporting	Providing feedback on performance relative to peers and public reporting of performance data motivate change in performance.
Patient-centered care, patient involvement, shared decision making	Patient autonomy and control over disease and care processes lead to better care and outcomes.
Total quality management and continuous quality improvement, restructuring processes, quality systems, breakthrough projects	Improving care comes from changing the systems, not from changing individuals.

Source: Adapted from Grol, R. (2001).

length of stay in intensive care units (Brook et al., 1999). Nevertheless, significant barriers exist to implementing EBP and using evidence-based clinical practice guidelines, including a lack of awareness that the guidelines exist, a lack of agreement, and a lack of ability to implement the guidelines (Cabana et al., 1999). As a result, efforts to implement guidelines are often not successful, and improvements in the processes of care have been disappointing (Bero et al., 1998; Grol & Grimshaw, 1999). In addition, few studies have evaluated the impact of EBP or evidence-based guidelines on patient outcomes.

Professional Education and Development

Professional education and development strategies address the complexity of clinical practice and propose improvement based on professional self-regulation and ownership by clinicians (Grol, 2001). Although classic continuing education approaches have been shown to be relatively ineffective, new approaches resembling simulation, including interactive forms of education and small group learning, have been effective for changing clinical performance (Davis et al., 1999). Nevertheless, additional research is needed to evaluate the cost-effectiveness of these new approaches because they require significant resources for implementation and maintenance (Grol, 2001).

Regular Assessments of Clinical Performance and Public Accountability

A third approach to improving quality of care emphasizes regular assessments of clinical performance and public accountability. The assumption is that providers will change practice when their performance is compared to their peers or presented for others to see. This approach is popular among purchasers, insurers, regulators, and accrediting bodies (www.jcaho.org; www.qualityforum.org). Providers, however, have concerns regarding the reliability and validity of the quality measures used. Consequently, this approach has done little to improve overall performance in health care to date (Chassin & Galvin, 1998; Thomson et al., 1999).

Patient-Centered Care

Patient-centered care emphasizes the need to empower patients to participate in medical decision making. Methods employed include patient satisfaction surveys, complaint procedures, needs assessments, decision aids, and risk tables for "shared decision making" (Grol, 2001). In critical care, for example, several validated tools are now available for evaluating patient and family satisfaction (Heyland & Tranmer, 2001; Wasser et al., 2001). Whether or how these data change performance is less clear. Moreover, patients' desire to participate in care varies among cultures. Given the complexity of patient care, it is unlikely that a single empowerment method will be generalizable across different settings, different patient populations, and different situations.

Total Quality Management

Total quality management (TQM) and continuous quality improvement (CQI) propose an integrated approach to improving patient care. TQM and CQI emphasize that the greatest opportunity for improvement is found by focusing on the health system's organizational characteristics rather than on individuals. In TQM, providers measure performance, change what they do, and evaluate the impact of that change.

Performance Improvement through Measurement

The underlying principle for all of these approaches is that if we want to improve the quality of care that we provide, providers must be able to measure their performance. Nevertheless, healthcare providers have limited ability to obtain feedback regarding performance in their daily work, due in part to a lack of information systems and to a lack of agreement on how to measure quality of care (McGlynn & Ashe, 1998). As a result, many of us in health care do not have access to performance data and, consequently, do not know the results we are achieving (or failing to achieve). For example, if asked what our nosocomial infection rate is or our average duration of mechanical ventilation, many of us may not know.

We need to train all members of the healthcare team in the methodology of improvement. The quality improvement model developed by Nolan is the most widely accepted, yet, in our experience, few healthcare professionals are aware of this important conceptual model. Nolan's model includes a reflective component and an active component (Berwick, 1996). The reflective component seeks to identify aims and measures, and to change strategies by asking: What is our goal? How will we know when we reach our goal? What changes will we make to achieve our goal? The active component uses learning cycles to plan and test changes in systems and processes that usually are referred to as Plan-Do-Study-Act (PDSA) cycles. This quality improvement model attempts to analyze and improve processes, initially testing the change on a small scale prior to wide dissemination. It is described in further detail in Chapter 4.

Patient Safety as a Measure of Healthcare Quality

Safe care is the first of six aims for improving healthcare quality identified in the IOM (2001) report. The underlying premise of this aim is that patients should not be harmed by the care that is intended to help them. "First, do no harm," the ancient maxim that has grounded the practice of medicine since its earliest days, has put the safety of patients first and foremost in the minds of healthcare practitioners. Adverse events usually result in harm. We know that complications cause increased mortality (Figure 1.2). We also know that complications result in increased cost (Figure 1.3). Therefore, it is not surprising that safety heads the list of quality improvement aims.

A key assumption of this primary aim is that safety is a system property, rather than a characteristic of individuals. In order to reduce risk and ensure safety, clinicians must focus on designing systems that help prevent errors, or that mitigate harm from those errors that cannot be entirely prevented.

Successful error reduction has some common themes. Table 1.2 describes basic error reduction techniques. Any one of these techniques could result in an implementation plan with baseline measures, implementation of change, and remeasurement through a PDSA framework. One technique is to simplify care. This can be done by reducing the number of steps in the workflow process. For example, implementation of a provider order entry system that interfaces with the pharmacy system and the nursing medication administration record could eliminate the manual transcription step and the need to transmit orders via facsimile, both of which can lead to medication error. Another technique is to encourage voluntary reporting of errors and hazardous conditions. We cannot measure what we do not know.

Figure 1.2 Complications Increase Mortality

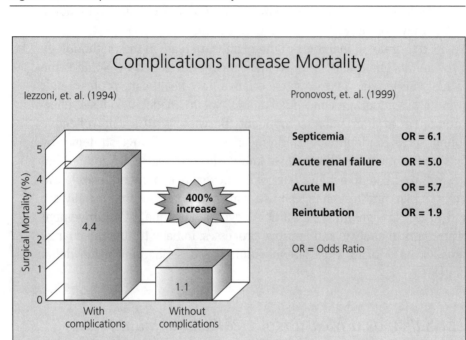

Figure 1.3 Complications Increase Cost

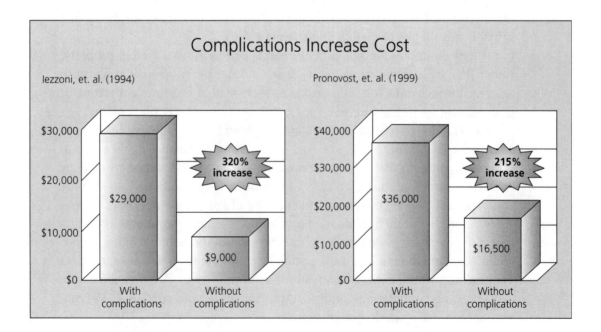

Table 1.2 Concepts of Error Reduction

1. Simplify
2. Standardize
3. Stratify
4. Improve auditory communication patterns
5. Support communication against the authority gradient
6. Use defaults properly
7. Automate cautiously
8. Use affordances and natural mapping
9. Respect limits on vigilance and attention
10. Encourage reporting of errors and hazardous conditions

Source: Adapted from Berwick, D. M. (1998).

Why Should Nurses Measure Safety Outcomes?

If you think about it, errors have always occurred in health care. We became tolerant of errors for a variety of reasons. One reason is that before the publication of the IOM (1999) report on medical errors, we the public did not understand the magnitude of the safety problem. We needed a measure, or quality metric, to understand the effect of our tolerance.

In this book, measuring safety outcomes allows us to quantify attributes of structures and processes that protect patients from injury, and the favorable or adverse effects these attributes have on patient health. Nurses are an essential member of the safety improvement team, and contribute their assessment of the work environment and knowledge of the work process utilized to administer care. Articulating this firsthand knowledge helps others on the team understand the intricate processes in the delivery of care. When a surgeon is ready to make an incision, hundreds of processes have occurred that must be 100% accurate, or an error can occur. These processes include admitting the patient under the right name (admitting), choosing the correct patient in the computer when blood is drawn for a type and crossmatch (laboratory), validation of consents (physician and nurse), preparing the correct instruments (central sterile, nurses, and technicians), making sure the equipment is in proper order (biomedical engineering), and posting the case properly (physician office staff and posting). This list is by no means inclusive and is an example of the complexity of the system, a system that must be redesigned for safety. There are many reasons the nurses should be engaged in these efforts to build safe systems.

The urgency of providing safe environments for patients is supported through the nurse's professional commitment to providing nursing services for patients (ANA, 2001). This professional commitment is built on the respect for human dignity, and the nurse's dedication to protect and preserve life. In protecting patients from harm through safety initiatives, nurses can directly reduce the risk of injury.

Professional organizations have focused education, tools, and resources on safety for their members. One example, The Association for periOperative Registered Nurses (AORN), has created a "Patient Safety First" initiative, which provides a wide variety of information for members (AORN, 2004).

So, why should nurses measure safety? The basic tenet is that safety is an important priority, not only from the national policy or organizational perspective, but also from the personal perspectives of nurses who work with individual patients. Nurses can have a direct effect on the safety of patients both individually and in teams by identifying opportunities for improving work processes.

Conclusion

This chapter has introduced the concept of patient safety as it relates to healthcare quality. Patient safety is a major priority to patients, healthcare professionals, organizations, and policy makers. Safety is a basic component of healthcare quality. Nurses are integral to the discovery and correction of vulnerable processes that can harm the patient. This discovery and correction is dependent on a transformed work environment in health care with an appropriate organizational culture and leadership. Nurses are essential members of the team that builds safe care processes. Achieving skill in measuring patient safety is a foundational building block.

References

American Nurses Association. (2001). *Code of ethics for nurses with interpretive statements*. Washington, DC: American Nurses Publishing.

Angus, D. C., Kelley, M. A., Schmitz, R. J., White, A., Popovich, J., et al. (2000). Current and projected workshop requirements for the care of the critically ill patient and patients with pulmonary disease: Can we meet the requirements of an aging population? *Journal of the American Medical Association, 284,* 2762–2770.

AORN. (2004). *Patient Safety First from AORN*. Retrieved June 2, 2004, from http://www.patientsafetyfirst.org.

Bero, L. A., Grilli, R., Grimshaw, J. M., Harvey, E., Oxman, A. D., Thomson, M. A. (1998). Closing the gap between research and practice: An overview of systematic reviews of interventions to promote the implementation of research findings. The Cochrane Effective Practice and Organization of Care Review Group. *British Journal of Medicine, 317,* 465–8.

Berwick, D. M. (1996). Harvesting knowledge from improvement. *Journal of the American Medical Association, 275,* 877–8.

Berwick, D. M. (1998). Examining errors in health care. Developing a prevention, education, and research agenda. Presentation to American Hospital Association Centennial Regional Leadership Forum, Cleveland, Ohio, June 24, 1998. Retrieved July 10, 2003, from http://www.ihi.org/resources/patientsafety/presentations/

Blumenthal, D. (1996). Part 1: Quality of care—what is it? *New England Journal of Medicine, 335,* 891–894.

Brook, R. H., McGlynn, E. A., & Cleary, P. D. (1997). Quality of health care. Part 2: Measuring quality of care. *New England Journal of Medicine, 336,* 804, discussion 806–807.

Cabana, M. D., Rand, C. S., Powe, N. R., Wu, A. W., Wilson, M. H., Abboud, P. A., Rubin, H. R. (1999). Why don't physicians follow clinical practice guidelines? A framework for improvement. *Journal of the American Medical Association, 282,* 1458–65.

Chassin, M. R., & Galvin, R. W. (1998). The urgent need to improve health care quality. Institute of Medicine National Roundtable on Health Care Quality. *Journal of the American Medical Association, 280,* 1000–1005.

Clermont, G., Angus, D. C., DiRusso, S. M., Griffin, M., & Linde-Zwirble, W. T. (2001). Predicting hospital mortality for patients in the intensive care unit: A comparison of artificial neural networks with logistic regression models, *Critical Care Medicine, 29,* 291–296.

Davis, D., O'Brien, M. A., Freemantle, N., Wolf, F. M., Mazmanian, P., Taylor-Vaisey, A. (1999). Impact of formal continuing medical education: Do conferences, workshops, rounds, and other traditional continuing education activities change physician behavior or health care outcomes? *Journal of the American Medical Association, 282,* 867–74.

Grol, R., Grimshaw, J. (1999). Evidence-based implementation of evidence-based medicine. *The Joint Commission Journal on Quality Improvement, 10,* 503–13.

Grol, R. (2001). Improving the quality of medical care: Building bridges among professional pride, payor profit, and patient satisfaction. *Journal of the American Medical Association, 286,* 2578–2585.

Heyland, D. K., Tranmer, J. E., Kingston General Hospital ICU Research Working Group. (2001). Measuring family satisfaction with care in the intensive care unit: The development of a questionnaire and preliminary results. *Journal of Critical Care, 4,* 142–9.

Iezzoni, L. I., Daley, J. , Heeren, T., Foley, S. M., Fisher, E. S., Duncan, C., Hughes, J. S., & Coffman, G. A. (1994). Identifying complications of care using administrative data. *Medical Care, 32,* 700–715.

Institute of Medicine. (1999). *To err is human: Building a better health care system.* Washington, DC: National Academy Press.

Institute of Medicine. (2001). *Crossing the quality chasm: A new health system for the 21st century.* Washington, DC: National Academy Press.

Institute of Medicine. (2003). *IOM definition of quality.* Retrieved July 9, 2003, from http:///www.iom.edu.

Institute of Medicine. (2004). *Keeping patients safe: Transforming the work environment for nurses.* Washington, DC: National Academy Press.

Leape, L. (2000). Institute of Medicine medical error figures are not exaggerated. *Journal of the American Medical Association, 284,* 95–97.

Leape, L. L., Cullen, D. J., Clapp, M. D., Burdick, E., Demonaco, H. J., Erickson, J. I., & Bates, D. W. (1999). Pharmacist participation on physician rounds and adverse drug events in the intensive care unit, *Journal of the American Medical Association, 282,* 267–270.

McGlynn, E. A. (1998). Choosing and evaluating clinical performance measures. *Joint Commission Journal on Quality Improvement, 24,* 470–479.

McGlynn, E.A. (2003). Selecting common measures of quality and system performance. *Medical Care, 41*(1, Supplement), I-39–I-47.

McGlynn, E. A., & Ashe, S. M. (1998). Developing a clinical performance measure. *American Journal of Preventive Medicine, 14*(3Suppl), 14–21.

President's Advisory Commission on Consumer Protection and Quality in the Health Care Industry. (1998). *Quality first: Better health care for all Americans.* Silver Springs, MD: Agency for Health Care Research and Quality Publications Clearinghouse.

Pronovost, P. J., Dang, D., Dorman, T., Lipsett, P. A., Garrett, E., Jenckes, M., & Bass, E. B. (2001). Intensive care unit nurse staffing and the risk for complications after abdominal aortic surgery. *Effective Clinical Practice, 4,* 199–206.

Pronovost, P. J., Jenckes, M. W., Dorman, T., Garrett, E., Breslow, M. J., Rosenfeld, B. A., Lipsett, P. A., & Bass, E. (1999). Organizational characteristics of intensive care units related to outcomes of abdominal aortic surgery. *Journal of the American Medical Association, 281,* 1310–1317.

Reeder, J. M. (2002). *Patient safety: Competency assessment module.* Denver, CO: Certification Boards.

Sackett, D. L., Rosenberg, W. M., Gray, J. A., Haynes, R. B., Richardson, W. S. (1996). Evidence based medicine: What it is and what it isn't. *British Journal of Medicine, 312,* 71–72.

Thomson, M., Oxman, A., Davis, D., et al. (1999). Audit and feedback to improve health professional practice and health care outcomes [Cochrane Review on CD-ROM]. *Cochrane Review,* 1.

Wasser, T., Pasquale, M. A., Matchett, S. C., Bryan, Y., Pasquale, M. (2001). *Critical Care Medicine, 1,* 192–6.

Zimmerman, J. E., Wagner, D. P., Draper, E. A., Wright, L., Alzola, C., & Knaus, W. A. (1998). Evaluation of acute physiology and chronic health evaluation III: Predictions of hospital mortality in an independent database. *Critical Care Medicine, 26,* 1317–1326.

CHAPTER 2

Using Performance Improvement to Support Patient Safety

Stephanie S. Poe, MScN, RN*

Y ou walk into Mrs. Benton's room at the start of your shift to make an initial assessment of her condition. As you perform a check of her multiple intravenous lines, you note that the rate on the fentanyl intravenous pump is much higher than the prescribed rate. Although the patient had been ordered to receive 25 mcg fentanyl per hour, the pump was set to deliver 250 mcg fentanyl per hour. Immediately you correct the pump settings to the prescribed rate. Luckily, the patient exhibits no hemodynamic compromise, but you know that this event had the potential to cause significant harm. You are aware that incorrect pump programming happens quite frequently and have read about "smart" pumps that can help to prevent these types of errors. You sigh and remember that it is difficult to get the hospital to commit to any new purchases, much less one that would require an entire fleet replacement. If only you knew how a nurse clinician could bring about change in a complex organization!

Faced with the day-to-day challenges of an unpredictable, highly complex patient care environment, nurses often wonder how they can maintain the safety of their patients for the duration of a single shift, much less throughout the entire episode of care. Large work loads, high patient acuity, inexperienced staff, constant interruption, multiple hand-offs, time pressures, and fuzzy boundaries among disciplines all converge into a perfect setup for errors. Even when they identify potential areas for safety improvement, nurses find themselves

*The Johns Hopkins Hospital
 Baltimore, Maryland

speculating that the system in which they work is too immense for change. They perceive many organizational barriers to change, and therefore, are reluctant to try to act as change agents.

It is important for nurses to remember that everyone has a circle of influence. There will always be things that no one can change, just as there will always be things that you can fix all by yourself. Patient safety initiatives, on the other hand, are built on the premise that there are things you can change with the help of your colleagues, your supervisors, and the leadership of your organization.

The overall aim of this chapter is to provide clinical nurse leaders, educators, and managers with an understanding of how organizational performance improvement (PI) structures and processes can be used to support patient safety initiatives. The objectives are to:

- Discuss how the organization has codified safety principles
- Link PI structures and processes with internally and externally driven patient safety priorities
- Describe how PI enables staff nurses to actively participate in interdisciplinary patient safety projects
- Explore methods to develop and communicate measures of success

The chapter will close with recommendations for nurse leaders to successfully integrate patient safety into PI programs with the overall goal of quality and safety in patient care.

Codification of Safety Principles

A key element in successful patient safety programs is the codification of safety principles; that is, the creation of policies based on ethical and clinical principles and using internal and external cues to catalyze staff-driven evidence-based policy reform (Nursing Executive Center [NEC], 2003). An organization's PI program is guided by its mission and values. Ensuring that its mission and value set clearly establish patient safety as an imperative allows the organization to outwardly communicate its commitment to the Hippocratic maxim "do no harm." Values intrinsic to the safety mission statement should build on the organization's code of ethics. Principles such as respect for persons, beneficence (maximizing benefits and minimizing harm), and justice are key patient safety values.

As nurse leaders begin to plan how to maximize the role of nurses in patient safety, they should teach nurses about how patient safety has been codified in their organization. For example, the three-part mission of our organization has long been patient care, education, and research. Therefore, a safety mission statement was written, based on this purpose: "The Johns Hopkins Hospital strives for safety in patient care, teaching and research" (JHH, 2002). In addition, an Ethical Framework for Safety (Williams & Rushton, 2002) was developed that identifies other important supporting values, including humility, honesty, and fidelity (the underpinnings of error disclosure) and diligence and learning (the essentials of continual identification and response to actual or potential threats to patient safety). An introduction to these two documents is part of every nurse's orientation, and key components are included in annual review packets for current nursing staff.

Putting a safety mission statement and its attendant values into words is relatively easy; translating them into action directed toward improving the structures and processes of care is more difficult. Creating and communicating evidence-based standards that incorporate patient safety values and lessons learned through safety-focused improvement projects is one way to accomplish this transformation. By using information generated by reports of internal and external adverse events to drive evidence-based policy reform, a perpetual safety-improvement cycle can be created (NEC, 2003). This information will be more credible when leaders succinctly communicate progress through goal-directed process and outcome measures. This information exchange should include all disciplines, because patient care does not occur in isolation. In addition, two-way communication should occur with all levels of staff, because those who do the work of patient care are in the best position to identify ways to improve patient safety.

Information gleaned from internal risk screening mechanisms (adverse event reports, computer-generated triggers or alerts, informal stories shared by staff) can be used to generate policy change. Additionally, recommendations following analysis of external events by credible sources can also drive change. One prominent source of such analyses is The Joint Commission on Accreditation of Healthcare Organizations (JCAHO), which publishes periodic *Sentinel Event Alerts* to share the most important lessons learned—known risky behaviors as well as best practice recommendations—from its database of error-related information (O'Leary, 2000). Over the years, the JCAHO has issued alerts in a number of areas, including medication errors, wrong site surgery, restraint-related deaths, blood transfusion errors, inpatient suicides, infant abductions, and post-operative complications. Another evidence-based source of medication-related events and best practice recommendations is the Institute of Safe Medication Practices (ISMP), which publishes the *ISMP Medication Safety Alert!* (ISMP, 2003).

Alignment of Safety and Performance Improvement

In 2001, revisions that directly link PI and safety appeared in the "Improving Organization Performance" chapter in the *Comprehensive Accreditation Manual for Hospitals: The Official Handbook (CAMH)* (JCAHO, 2001). These standards advise leaders to consider safety when designing processes, functions, or services; address safety issues when collecting data to monitor performance; and set priorities and assign responsibility for proactive risk identification and reduction (Joint Commission Resources, 2002).

Another key element in successful patient safety programs is institution of a staff-centered safety infrastructure, including training programs targeted to address safety weaknesses, rapid-action safety committees, and open-door meetings (NEC, 2003). By weaving patient safety into the fabric of existing PI committee structures and creating new structures where holes are identified, the organization can configure these structures to prioritize safety-focused opportunities for improvement.

Nurses at all levels of the organization need an understanding of how patient safety is integrated into existing PI structures. An example of the seamless integration of safety and PI structures can be seen in Figure 2.1. This figure depicts the JHH PI committee structure, and reflects communication lines leading from the bedside clinician up to the board of trustees, as well as integration with the medical board committee structure. The PI council serves as a steering committee, and receives recommendations and reports from its subcommittees. These subcommittees include groups charged with regulatory compliance, clinical PI, service PI, departmental PI (encompassing all clinical departments, including nursing), and patient safety. Each of these subcommittees receives reports and recommendations from all levels of unit- and department-based staff. In addition, the PI committee structure has a direct link to the administrative committee of the medical board through the patient safety committee.

Figure 2.1   The Johns Hopkins Hospital Performance Improvement Committee Structure

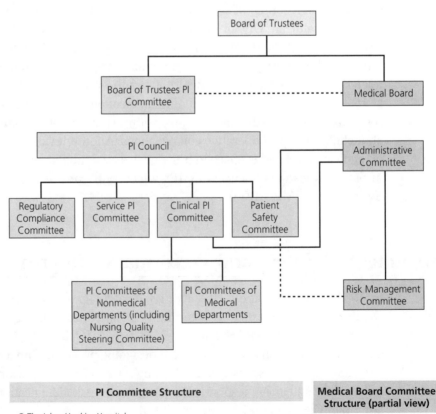

© The Johns Hopkins Hospital

Based on staff input, the JHH PI council set three organizational goals for improvement in 2003, one of which was patient safety. Each subcommittee oversees or serves as a clearinghouse for a variety of interdisciplinary safety-focused PI initiatives carried out by units throughout the hospital, many of which are led by nursing. Examples of such unit- or department-based initiatives are illustrated in subsequent chapters.

Enabling Staff Participation

Given the complexity of the healthcare delivery system and the ever-growing demands placed on staff working within that system, enabling staff participation is a challenge. This is particularly true of nurses, in light of persistent staff shortages. W. Edwards Deming long ago postulated that workers work in a system and that the job of the manager is to work on the system with the workers' help (Tribus, n.d.). Who can better determine which fixes would achieve a safer system than the workers who function within that inherently flawed system on a day-to-day basis? If organizational leadership is truly committed to staff involvement in developing innovations, measuring outcomes, and making recommendations for application of best practices to ensure a model patient safety system, then its leaders must dedicate resources to make it happen.

It is important to build a broad base of support for PI and safety initiatives. By providing personnel, training, information system support, coaches, tools, and technology, an organization can help "to build a grass-roots enterprise that turns to physicians, nurses and managers to gather data, evaluate changes, and recommend best practices" (Miller, 2002). Such an organization support structure was developed at our institution. This structure has identified several challenges for 2004, two of which are safety-focused (no harm from infection and no harm by medication error), and has supported a variety of safety improvement projects. Examples of such projects include efforts seeking to reduce the risk of:

- catheter-related bloodstream, cardiac coronary artery bypass graft, and laminectomy surgical site infections
- adverse events related to anticoagulation, patient-controlled analgesia, and chemotherapy
- missing medication doses

Priority Performance Improvement Topics

Frequently identified safety-focused performance improvement issues include measures related to sentinel events and patient safety goals, hospital-acquired infection, medication safety, and nurse-sensitive safety measures. Each of these topics will be further discussed in the following sections.

Sentinel Events and Patient Safety Goals

Safety-focused performance measures are often developed in response to external regulatory forces. Two such outcome measures regularly monitored at the JHH include "number of sentinel events" and "number of repeated sentinel events." A sentinel event is defined as: "an unexpected occurrence involving death or serious physical or psychological injury or the risk thereof. *Serious injury* specifically includes loss of limb or function. The phrase '*or the risk thereof*' includes any process variation for which a recurrence would carry a significant chance of a serious adverse outcome" (JHH, 2003).

In 2001, as a direct result of its work related to sentinel events, the JCAHO introduced national Patient Safety Goals that will be modified on a yearly basis. The Sentinel Event Advisory Group reviewed reported sentinel events for recommendations from root cause analyses, identified critical initiatives to improve patient safety, and developed national Patient Safety Goals (JCAHO, 2002). Acute care hospitals are required to implement the best practice recommendations accompanying each goal. The 2004 JCAHO Patient Safety Goals, best practice recommendations, and sample process and outcome measures are included in Table 2.1. Nursing staff should be aware of these goals, and should be actively involved in patient safety initiatives directed toward the achievement of these goals.

Hospital-Acquired Infection

The most common complications affecting hospitalized patients today are hospital-acquired, or nosocomial, infections, and the need for renewed commitment to and innovations in infection prevention to help ensure patient safety is clear (Burke, 2003). Historically examined through the lens of epidemiology, infection surveillance activities are critical components of patient safety. Infection control experts advocate viewing each infection as potentially preventable (unless proven otherwise) and recommend that infections trigger closer scrutiny of the safety and appropriateness of medical treatment (Gerberding, 2002).

There is no doubt that infection prevention and control is a major patient safety concern. The rate of hospital-acquired infections per 1,000 patient days increased 36% from 7.2 in 1975 to 9.8 in 1995, accounting for approximately 88,000 deaths (Weinstein, 1998). Urinary catheter–associated urinary tract infection (UTI), central-line associated bloodstream infection (BSI), surgical site infection, and ventilator-associated pneumonia account for most nosocomial infections, with 25% of these occurring in ICU environments and 70% due to antimicrobial–resistant microorganisms (Burke, 2003). Therefore, many hospitals monitor the following device-associated outcome measures as part of their ICU safety-focused infection control surveillance activities: urinary catheter–associated UTI rate (denominator = number of urinary catheter days), central line–associated BSI rate (denominator = number of central line days), ventilator-associated pneumonia rate (denominator = number of ventilator days), and surgical site infection rates. As a benchmark for comparison, The

Table 2.1 JCAHO 2004 Patient Safety Goals*, Recommendations*, and Sample Metrics

Patient Safety Goal	Recommendations	Sample Metrics
Goal 1: Improve the accuracy of patient identification	Use at least two patient identifiers whenever taking blood samples or administering medications or blood products.	Reported errors related to blood samples, blood product, or medication administration involving misidentification
	Before starting any surgical or invasive procedure, conduct an active final verification process (e.g., a "time out") to confirm correct patient, procedure, and site.	Number of time out procedures observed or documented per surgical cases started
Goal 2: Improve the effectiveness of communication among caregivers	Implement a verification "read-back" process for verbal or telephone orders.	Reported medication errors related to verbal or telephone orders
	Standardize abbreviations, acronyms, and symbols used, including a list of prohibited acronyms, abbreviations, and symbols.	Number of times prohibited abbreviations appear in orders
Goal 3: Improve the safety of using high-alert medications	Remove concentrated electrolytes from patient care units.	Number of times restricted electrolytes are found during unit inspections
	Standardize and limit the number of available drug concentrations.	Reported medication errors involving wrong concentration
Goal 4: Eliminate wrong site, wrong patient, wrong procedure surgery	Use a preoperative verification process (e.g., checklist) to confirm that appropriate documents are available.	Number of times preoperative checklist is incomplete
	Implement a process to mark the surgical site, and involve patient in the marking.	Reported occurrences of wrong site, wrong patient, wrong procedure surgery
Goal 5: Improve the safety of using infusion pumps	Ensure free-flow protection on all general-use and PCA intravenous infusion pumps.	Reported medication errors involving free-flow
Goal 6: Improve the effectiveness of clinical alarm systems	Implement regular preventive maintenance and testing of alarm systems.	Reported inoperable alarm systems
	Assure that alarms are activated with appropriate settings and are sufficiently audible	Reported events where inaudible alarm was a contributing factor
Goal 7: Reduce the risk of healthcare-acquired infections	Comply with current CDC hand hygiene guidelines.	Observed use of alcohol-based gel hand rubs by direct caregivers
	Manage as sentinel events all identified cases of unanticipated death or major permanent loss of function associated with a healthcare-acquired infection.	Number of sentinel events associated with a healthcare-acquired infection

*Note: Adapted from Special Report! 2004 JCAHO National Patient Safety Goals: Practical Strategies and Helpful Solutions for Meeting These Goals. *Joint Commission Perspectives on Patient Safety, 3*(9),1–11.

National Nosocomial Infections Surveillance System of the U.S. Centers for Disease Control and Prevention collects data on all sites of nosocomial infection in patients located in ICUs, as well as ICU-specific denominator data (NNISS, 2002). Prior to January 1999, this system contained a hospital-wide component, which has since been eliminated due to time and resource constraints.

Handwashing, now more appropriately called hand hygiene, is a simple but fundamental clinical action for controlling nosocomial infections in patients (O'Boyle, Henly, & Duckett, 2001). The latest guidelines from the Centers for Disease Control recommend the following process measures for assessing improvements in hand-hygiene adherence (Boyce & Pittet, 2002):

- Number of hand-hygiene episodes performed by personnel/number of hand-hygiene opportunities, by ward or by service
- Volume of alcohol-based hand rub (or detergent used for handwashing or hand antisepsis) used per 1,000 patient-days
- Reported incidents of staff wearing artificial nails

Medication Safety

Addressing medication errors and near misses, known collectively as America's other drug problem, has become paramount in 21st century U.S. health care (Brown, 2001). The industry is constantly being bombarded with new technological applications that can provide medication safety nets. In order to determine whether technological solutions such as barcode-enabled point of care systems and computerized provider order entry would truly reduce harm from medication errors, appropriate process and outcome measures are essential.

Most organizations have some type of medication error reporting system that produces such outcome measures as medication errors per 10,000 billed doses or signification medication errors per 10,000 billed doses. Medication error rates related to prescription, transcription, dispensing, and administration are calculated and trends are reviewed.

The utility of tracking reported medication errors has been noted to be somewhat limited. The National Coordinating Council for Medication Error Reporting and Prevention (NCC-MERP) suggests that use of medication error rates is not a valid method to compare healthcare organizations due to variability in definitions and methods of calculation (NCC-MERP, 2002). Depending upon the organizational culture, calculated medication rates may be more an indicator of the culture of safety rather than an accurate measure of organizational performance (Combes, 2003); that is, the clinical area that has a large number of self-reports may be the unit that has the most highly developed culture of safety in which staff members have internalized the obligation to report errors. In contrast, staff on the clinical unit with the lowest reported rate may be reluctant to report due to fear of reprisal.

Internal trend analyses of medication errors and near misses are useful at the organizational level to identify potential areas of analysis for safety improvement opportunities. At the very least, they provide the added value of detecting safety opportunities at a more granular level. Such analyses may reveal that an organization has an increase in reporting of errors associated with intravenous infusion device programming when delivering such high-alert medications as narcotics, anticoagulants, high concentration electrolytes, or chemotherapies.

Communication of the finding from in-depth analyses of infusion pump errors has had the added advantage of making health care's industrial partners aware of opportunities to improve existing technologies. New "smart pumps" are now available with a wide array of built-in safety features (Eskew et al., 2002). Nurse leaders at JHH used data derived from our internal trend analyses to make the decision to invest limited resources in this new technology.

When changes are added to the medication system to make it safer, process measures can be identified that specifically test the effectiveness of these changes. For example, chemotherapy, with its narrow therapeutic index and complex treatment regimens, has the potential for significant harm if not administered as intended (Branowicki et al., 2003). To build a safer chemotherapy administration system at JHH, we implemented a new interdisciplinary chemotherapy protocol and an accompanying checklist to encourage collaborative validation of chemotherapy orders. We then identified various process measures to monitor compliance with the new processes we put into place.

Nurse-Sensitive Safety Measures

The American Nurses Association (ANA) has actively participated in efforts to measure patient safety for many years, including developing and testing nursing-sensitive patient outcome indicators (ANA, 1995; 1996). In the wake of the healthcare restructuring era of the 1990s, the ANA, as part of its Safety and Quality Initiative, has been very vocal about the increased risks to patients resulting from inadequate staffing. By linking nurse-sensitive outcomes to staffing levels and staff composition, it is hoped that nurse leaders will identify systems and processes to reduce risk of error. A phase 2 study of the nursing quality outcome indicators (specifically, nurse satisfaction, patient satisfaction, patient falls, and pressure ulcers) was undertaken in North Dakota, and findings indicated that examination of fall and pressure ulcer rates was useful in problem solving (Langemo, Anderson, & Volden, 2002).

In July 2002, the JCAHO implemented staffing effectiveness measures, designed to focus organizations on assessing the relationship between staffing and patient outcomes (JCAHO, 2001). These measures use an evidence-based model that includes human resource and clinical/service indicators. Suggested clinical measures felt to be potentially affected by staffing parameters included patient falls, adverse drug events, injuries to patients, skin breakdown, pneumonia, postoperative infection, UTI, upper gastrointestinal bleeding, and shock/cardiac arrest.

Communicating Successes

Certainly, performance on institutional safety measures should be communicated throughout all levels of the organization, from the bedside care provider to the board of trustees. In addition, recommendations for best practices that are generated as a result of institutional safety improvement projects should provide the basis for research studies designed to test their generalizability for improving safety at other institutions. Our organization maintains a close link between the nursing research and nursing performance improvement committees to enable collaboration in identifying potential areas for research.

Over the last decade, leading healthcare executives have begun to advocate for the use of monthly performance "dash boards" to give executives a user-friendly snapshot of a complex organization's overall performance (Health Care Advisory Board, 2000). By necessity, this type of visual report card should be balanced among the domains of interest to the organization. At our organization, a PI Profile is generated on a monthly basis. This profile contains measures reflecting performance on the following dimensions: clinical, service, fiscal, and infrastructure. Within the clinical domain, selected performance measures address safety and clinical effectiveness. Table 2.2 includes the subset of safety measures included on our PI Profile. These measures were based on organizational safety priorities.

Table 2.2 Safety Measures Included in the JHH Performance Improvement Profile

Clinical Patient Safety Performance Measures
Number of Sentinel Events
Number of Repeated Sentinel Events
Reported Significant Medication Errors
Patient Fall with Injury Rate
Number of Serious Injuries/Deaths Associated with a Device
Missing Medication Dose Rate
Device-Associated ICU Bloodstream Infection Rate
VRE (Vancomycin-Resistant Enterococci) Bloodstream Infection Rate
MRSA (Methicillin-Resistant Staph Aureus) Bloodstream Infection Rate
Pediatric Nosocomial RSV (Respiratory Synctival Virus) Rate
Nosocomial Influenza Rate

Recommendations for Nurse Leaders

Improvement in patient safety is achieved by clinicians, so nurses must have sound operational data on which to build capacity to improve (Galvin & McGlynn, 2003). According to Dickerson-Hazard (2003), capacity "is found not only in belief, desires and anticipated outcomes, but also in the currencies of time, talents, resources and knowledge." Nurses have valuable clinical and operational expertise that can contribute in significant ways to the design of innovative systems that reduce the risk of healthcare error.

Buerhaus (2003) identified three needs as top priorities for nursing knowledge to improve health (and therefore, patient safety): obtain good data on the relevant issue; develop skills to properly analyze the data; and develop skills to use the results of analyses, create a message, and communicate the message to all relevant parties. Active nurse leadership in outcome and process measure design will help ensure that nursing-sensitive patient outcomes and staffing effectiveness measures are included, as appropriate. This is especially true with respect to measuring safety outcomes.

Conclusion

This chapter has provided examples of how the performance improvement structures and processes within organizations can provide support for patient safety initiatives. Nurse leaders play an important role in identifying and addressing safety-focused organizational priorities, developing measures to assess overall system performance and patient safety, enabling staff nurse participation in safety improvement teams, and communicating results of these activities throughout all levels of the organization. With the help of such tools as codification of safety principles, integration of PI and safety structures and processes, and active participation of nurses in interdisciplinary safety improvement teams, nurse leaders are well-positioned to be key drivers of successful safety improvement programs.

References

American Nurses Association. (1995). *Nursing report card for acute care.* Washington, DC: American Nurses Publishing.

American Nurses Association. (1996). *Code nursing quality indicators: Definitions and implications.* Washington, DC: American Nurses Publishing.

American Nurses Association. (2001). *Code of ethics for nurses with interpretive statements.* Washington, DC: American Nurses Publishing.

Berwick, D. M., James, B., & Coye, M. J. (2003). Connections between quality measurement and improvement. *Medical Care, 41*(1, Supplement), I-30–I-38.

Boyce, J. M. & Pittet, D. (2002, October 25). Guideline for Hand Hygiene in Health-Care Settings: Recommendations of the Healthcare Infection Control Practices Advisory Committee and the HICPAC/SHEA/APIC/IDSA Hand Hygiene Task Force. *Morbidity and Mortality Weekly Report, 51*(RR16), 1–44.

Branowicki, P., O'Neill, J. B., Dwyer, J. L., Marino, B. L., Houlahan, K., & Billett, A. (2003). Improving complex medication systems. An interdisciplinary approach. *Journal of Nursing Administration, 33*, 199–200.

Brown, M. M. (2001). Managing medication errors by design. *Critical Care Nurse Quarterly 24*, 77–97.

Buerhaus, P. (2002). Priorities for advancing nursing knowledge. *Journal of Nursing Scholarship, 34*(3), 211–212.

Burke, J. P. (2003). Infection control—A problem for patient safety. *The New England Journal of Medicine, 348*, 651–656.

Combes, J. R. (2003). Comparing hospital performance by measuring medication error rates: Is it possible? *Focus on Patient Safety, 6*, 1–2.

Dickerson-Hazard, N. (2003, Second Quarter). 'See you at some ballgame, meeting or another!' *Reflections on Nursing Leadership*, 6.

Eskew, J. A., Jacobi, J., Buss, W. F., Warhurst, H. M., & DeBord, C. L. (2002). Using innovative technologies to set new safety standards for the infusion of intravenous medications. *Hospital Pharmacy, 37*, 1179–1189.

Galvin, R. S., & McGlynn, E. A. (2003).Using performance measurement to drive improvement: A road map for change. *Medical Care, 41*(1, Supplement), I-48–I-60.

Gerberding, J. L. (2002). Hospital-onset infections: A patient safety issue. *Annals of Internal Medicine, 137*, 665–670.

Health Care Advisory Board. (2000). *CEO dashboards. Performance metrics for the new health care economy*. Washington, DC: The Advisory Board Company.

Institute of Medicine. (1999). *To err is human: Building a better health care system*. Washington, DC: National Academy Press.

Institute of Medicine. (2001). *Crossing the quality chasm: A new health system for the 21st century*. Washington, DC: National Academy Press.

Institute of Safe Medication Practices. (2003). *ISMP Medication Safety Alert!* Retrieved May 1, 2003, from http://www.ismp.org

Johns Hopkins Hospital. (2002). Ethical framework for safety. In: *The Johns Hopkins Hospital Interdisciplinary clinical practice manual*. Baltimore, MD: The Johns Hopkins Hospital.

Johns Hopkins Hospital. (2003). MEL014 Sentinel event policy. In: *The Johns Hopkins Hospital interdisciplinary clinical practice manual*. Baltimore, MD: The Johns Hopkins Hospital.

The Joint Commission for Accreditation of Healthcare Organizations. (2001). *Comprehensive accreditation manual for hospitals: The official handbook (CAMH)*. Oakbrook Terrace, IL: JCAHO.

Joint Commission Resources. (2001). Using the new staffing effectiveness standards to improve safety. *Joint Commission Perspectives on Patient Safety, 1*(6), 1, 3, 5.

Joint Commission Resources. (2002). Standards link: Performance improvement and safety. *Joint Commission Perspectives on Patient Safety, 2*(7), 2.

Joint Commission Resources. (2002). Sentinel event alert advisory group identifies JCAHO's national patient safety goals. *Joint Commission Perspectives on Patient Safety, 2*(9), 1,3.

Langemo, D. K., Anderson, J., & Volden, C. M. (2002). Nursing quality outcome indicators. The North Dakota study. *Journal of Nursing Administration, 32*, 98–105.

McGlynn, E. A. (2003). Selecting common measures of quality and system performance. *Medical Care, 41*(1, Supplement), I-39–I-47.

Miller, E. D. (2002, Fall). Good outcomes take good systems. *Hopkins Medical News*. Retrieved May 1, 2003, from www.hopkinsmedicine.org/hmn/F02/postop.html

National Coordinating Council for Medication Error Reporting and Prevention. (2002, June 11). *Use of medication error rate to compare health care organizations is of NO value*. Statement.

National Nosocomial Infections Surveillance (NNIS). (2002, August). *Data summary from January 1992 to June 2002. American Journal of Infection Control, 30*, 458–475.

Nursing Executive Center. (2003). *Profiles in patient safety*. Washington, D.C.: The Advisory Board Company.

O'Boyle, C. A., Henly, S. J., & Duckett, L. J. (2001). Nurses' motivation to wash their hands: A standardized measurement approach. *Applied Nursing Research, 4,* 136–145.

O'Leary, D. (2000, February 22). *Statement of the Joint Commission on Accreditation of Health-care Organizations before the Committee on Health, Education, Labor and Pensions, U.S. Senate and the Subcommittee on Labor, Health and Human Services, and Education of the Senate Committee on Appropriations.* Retrieved June 3, 2004, from www.access.gpo.gov/congress/senate

Pronovost, P. J., & Berenholtz, S. M. (2002). *A practical guide to measuring performance in the intensive care unit.* VHA 2002 Research Series Volume 2, Irving, TX: VHA Inc.

Tribus, M. (n.d.). Deming's Redefinition of Management. Retrieved May 1, 2003, from http://deming.ces.clemson.edu/pub/den/demingdefmgt.pdf

Weinstein, R. A. (1998). Nosocomial infection update. *Emerging Infectious Diseases, 4,* 416–420.

Williams, M., & Rushton, C. (2002). The Johns Hopkins Hospital ethical framework for patient safety. In: *The Johns Hopkins Hospital interdisciplinary clinical practice manual.* Baltimore, MD: The Johns Hopkins Hospital.

CHAPTER 3

Moving Forward: Planning a Safety Project

*Patricia B. Dawson, MSN, RN**

As the nurse manager of a 30-bed inpatient unit, you have become increasingly concerned about the frequency and variety of patient-care adverse events that have occurred on your unit within the past several months. Each event has required an enormous amount of time for investigation and discussion with the unit staff and other disciplines involved. You are noticing that the typical recommendations for counseling or more education are not the solution. You decide to discuss your concerns at the next interdisciplinary quality steering meeting. You begin to think about the process to plan a safety project and who should be involved.

Previous studies have revealed that a multitude of safety risks and adverse events occur in the hospital setting (Shojania, Wald, & Gross, 2002). One of the challenges facing managers, educators, and staff involved in safety projects is how to proceed with planning in order to implement a safety project. Questions arise such as: Who should be involved? How do you get the buy-in that is necessary to make the changes? What steps should be taken? What tools are available to facilitate the process? All of these questions and challenges can be answered by using the common five *senses* that are often used in day-to-day management and daily life. This chapter will provide practical information on applying an eight-step process for project planning and discuss the role of the nurse participating in safety projects. The overall aim of this chapter is to prepare nurses to lead a safety project by providing a structured approach for planning and implementation. The specific objectives of this chapter are:

---

*The Johns Hopkins Hospital

■ Describe the steps in planning a safety project

■ Discuss the role of the nurse as a member of the multidisciplinary safety team

Assumptions and Realities

Creating an environment and a culture that makes safety a priority will require some consensus building to lay the groundwork for change (Wong, Helsinger, & Petry, 2002). It will be important to address the myths and realities that are associated with this type of process in order to enlist the support of administration and engage nursing staff and other members of the multidisciplinary team.

Common assumptions held by the staff include misconceptions of the driving forces for safety changes, the resources required, and the temporary nature of safety projects. For example, a general perception may be that this safety initiative is just another project to satisfy some institutional requirement for an annual performance improvement project instead of an organizational commitment to the effort. Others may hold the belief that it is something a few staff members can do on their own, and they are powerless to change practice. The third myth is that this is a one-shot, limited project that is not related to a continuum of improvement.

The role of the manager or educator is to introduce a realistic vision that will promote a permanent focus on safety. Safety projects are not about satisfying an annual performance improvement project, but about building on the existing processes and programs of quality improvement (Mawjii et al., 2002). Done correctly, it is an iterative process of making adjustments and corrections along the way until the desired outcome is achieved each and every time. The program and the process must be nurtured or the positive resulting outcomes may disappear (Piotrowski & Hinshaw, 2002). Involvement in safety initiatives can be a beginning step toward changing the processes, attitudes, and behaviors of the staff. In addition to improving patient outcomes, involvement in safety initiatives can improve teamwork and energize staff (Bower, 2002).

A Comprehensive Patient Safety Program

A structured approach helps to frame the steps needed to conduct a safety project. A comprehensive patient safety program has been developed by a multidisciplinary team at Johns Hopkins, and then used to guide the planning and implementation of safety projects (Johns Hopkins University School of Medicine, 2002). The program includes an eight-step process (see Figure 3.1) that includes an assessment of the current climate, education of the staff, identification of safety concerns, an in-depth look at the problem, planning and implementation of improvement strategies, reviewing the progress, sharing the

Figure 3.1   Comprehensive Patient Safety Program

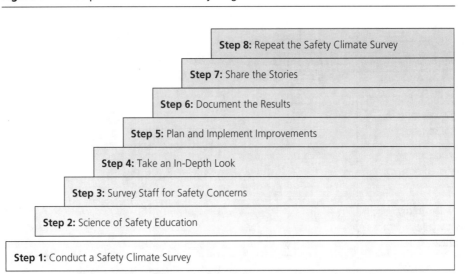

Adapted from Johns Hopkins School of Medicine, Baltimore, MD. © The Johns Hopkins Hospital

results, and resurveying staff. A common-sense approach can help the nurse leader to use his or her sense of touch, hearing, smell, and sight in the implementation of each of the eight steps of the process.

Step 1: Safety Climate Survey

The first step is to get a *feel* for the norms or beliefs of the unit or team. A framework for patient safety is built on the foundation of a cultural climate that allows clinicians to feel secure and blame-free in reporting errors. The environment must be perceived as conducive to developing improvements that will make the system better and protect against mistakes (Ketring & White, 2002; Piotrowski & Hinshaw, 2002). To know whether they have accomplished a culture shift through their safety project, the team must first assess the perceptions of the staff before they implement changes. This can be done through the administration of a climate survey. Our approach was to use a 19-item Likert scale questionnaire that could be completed by the respondent in less than 10 minutes (see Table 3.1). The survey responses help to identify staff perceptions of how important they believe safety is to the organization and to the unit. All interdisciplinary members who are a regular part of the unit operations and patient care activities (i.e., physicians, social workers, therapists, nurses, or unlicensed assistive personnel) should participate in the survey because the culture of the unit is affected by all individuals who interact with patients and staff. A more comprehensive version of this survey (Safety Attitudes Questionnaire) is available that provides a broader assessment of factors such as teamwork and collaboration. The longer version should be considered for use if there is significant buy-in and administrative support and the team anticipates

Table 3.1 Safety Climate Survey

	A	B	C	D	E	X
	Disagree Strongly	Disagree Slightly	Neutral	Agree Slightly	Agree Strongly	Not Applicable
1. The culture of this clinical area makes it easy to learn from the mistakes of others.						
2. Medical errors are handled appropriately in this clinical area.						
3. The senior leaders in my hospital listen to me and care about my concerns.						
4. The physician and nurse leaders in my areas listen to me and care about my concerns.						
5. Leadership is driving us to be a safety-centered institution.						
6. My suggestions about safety would be acted upon if I expressed them to management.						

Source: From Sexton et al., 2003. *Safety Climate Survey.* Used with permission courtesy of J. Bryan Sexton, PhD.

a long-lasting program or recurring projects (J. B. Sexton, personal communication, January 15, 2004).

Step 2: The Science of Safety Education

Following the survey, the staff needs to *hear* the facts and become better educated about the science of safety. This briefing should describe the magnitude of the problem and include stories about what others are doing to protect patients from the harms that exist in the typical healthcare setting. The education should prepare the staff for the reason that change is needed, how they can participate, and the importance of their participation. This session should begin to shift the focus away from the practitioner as the cause of problems and toward viewing safety problems from a systems approach. Collectively, as an interdisciplinary team, group members need to understand that traditional methods of blame, discipline, education, and policy writing cannot lead to the discovery of errors or flaws in a complex system of care (Ketring & White, 2002). The science of safety helps team members to appreciate and accept that human frailty exists, and that the goal is to look for the opportunity for error and then prevent it from happening or minimize the harm should it occur. Once this shift in thinking occurs, staff can become more analytical about the causes of safety problems and more creative about the potential solutions. The session is best viewed as a one-hour investment that will help to develop support for the action plans that will later be developed.

Step 3: Staff Survey

The next step involves an open-ended survey that seeks to *sniff out* the patient safety problems that staff members experience on a daily basis. The Institute of Medicine (IOM) report, *To Err Is Human: Building a Safer Health System* calls on health systems to focus more on error reduction as part of their regular operations (Maddox, Wakefield, & Bull, 2001). The survey is a first step toward answering this challenge, and it reinforces the lessons from the science of safety that error identification and prevention are a part of the new culture that should be promoted. The nurse leader is advised to avoid jumping to conclusions about what the safety issues are and what the priorities should be. The traditional hierarchy of decision making and priority setting will do little to promote the culture of a learning organization that will be needed in order to promote systems thinking and safer practices. Staff must believe and trust that their participation in any safety initiative is not an attempt to judge their competence. Soliciting their input to find areas for improvement can help to gain the trust that will be vital to the effort's success (Piotrowski & Hinshaw, 2002). In addition, the staff should be encouraged to offer suggestions on how processes or the environment could be changed to prevent or minimize the safety risks. The survey should be promoted as an opportunity to empower the staff/team to make a difference in patient care. They should be told that the information collected through this survey will be the basis for identifying and prioritizing the initiatives the unit will address.

The problems selected for action should be chosen on the basis of the potential for harm, the frequency of occurrence, the likelihood that an intervention could be developed and implemented, and the resources required to make the necessary change. The options need to be weighted by priority to make the decision of what to work on first. Having staff provide input into problem identification will promote their participation in problem solving.

Step 4: Taking an In-Depth Look

Once the specific safety initiative is identified, an interdisciplinary team should be assembled to take a critical *look* at the current system and processes of care. Redesigning care to incorporate safer practices can be complex due to the multiple providers and steps in the process. Careful attention must be given to the team's selection and support, as well as to the process of problem solving.

Successful experience with safety initiatives can be attributed not only to organizational and leadership support, but also to the presence of active support given to the project team. Three roles to be considered are those of champion, project leader or facilitator, and data analyst (Mawji et al., 2002). The champion, often an experienced clinician or respected administrator, is an individual who is recognized as an authority on the issue and can be influential in gaining approval and support for needed changes. A powerful strategy in demonstrating this type of support is the implementation of an Executive Adopt a Unit program. In this strategy, a senior hospital administrator adopts a unit and, through monthly team meetings, helps to identify and address safety issues. This individual is instrumental in helping the team to overcome barriers to the implementation of their plan (Johns Hopkins University School of Medicine, 2002). The project leader or facilitator assists the team by managing the project goals, objectives, timelines, and meeting agendas. The data analyst can facilitate the process of data collection and conversion of these data into information that will allow the team to track their progress.

The knowledge required to build safety into the system cannot be gained without the help of the clinicians who are most familiar with the process. Each discipline provides a piece of the safety puzzle and is a key stakeholder that must be included in the project. The Pittsburgh Regional Healthcare Initiative coalition set forth an objective to deliver perfect patient care. By adapting concepts from the Toyota Production System and the Alcoa Business System, they created a system in which the people actually performing the work solve the problems, measure the change, and share the results. In this design, the solutions are generated from the bottom up, and managers become partners in the process (Feinstein, Grunden, & Harrison, 2002). Participation should be voluntary, and it is helpful to include those individuals who can promote a sense of optimism about the potential for success in improving the system.

Once the team has been assembled, they should seek to gain a clear description of the threat or problem by exploring the facts that are available. The tendency of most teams is to plow forward and attempt to generate solutions for the perceived problem. In doing so, the team may be taking a short-sighted approach and fail to understand the true cause of the safety threat or problem. Worse yet, the group may lose valuable time and energy, only to find that each individual has a different perception of the defined problem. The basic knowledge needed includes: What does the problem look like when it happens? When does it typically occur and how often? Who is involved? After gathering these data, a structured process of analyzing the event will allow an objective examination of the process and system.

This objective examination by the team involves probing further to consider various factors that prevent the process from working as it should, creating a safety threat. A framework (see Table 3.2) for evaluating contributing factors to safety events can include an assessment of patient factors, task factors, individual factors, team factors, working conditions, and organization and management factors (Pronovost, Wu, Dorman, & Morlock, 2002). Each of these factors should be reviewed to determine whether it contributes to the safety problem and whether it represents an improvement opportunity.

Table 3.2   Framework for Assessing Contributing Factors

Factor	Criteria to Consider
Patient	Comorbidities and medical complexity Ability to communicate and comply Cultural issues
Task	Structure and design of process Availability of resources Accuracy of results
Individual	Training and education Physical and mental health
Team	Communication—written and verbal Delineation of tasks Supervision of assignments
Work conditions	Adequacy of staffing and support Maintenance of the environment and equipment
Organization and management	Goals and priorities Standards and policies

Source: Adapted from Pronovost, Wu, Dorman, & Morlock, 2002.

A frequent contributing factor to safety problems in today's healthcare environment is communication. The clarity of the plan of care is affected by factors such as whether the plan is communicated verbally, in writing, or both; whether the patient and/or family is included; and the number of hand-offs that can occur in the patient's care. Compound these factors with the decreasing length of stay and high technology in the current environment, and it is little wonder that communication is an often cited source of safety problems. While reviewing contributing factors in-depth, the team should be aware that several factors may be present in any given problem, and each of the factors should be reviewed before strategizing intervention solutions.

Step 5: Plan and Implement Improvements

Once the interdisciplinary team has taken an in-depth look at the possible contributing factors, they can begin to develop implementation strategies to anticipate and prevent errors, or to minimize the potential for harm. The action plan should include a *shared vision* of goals that are simple, focused, and measurable. Measurement criteria of the project's process and outcome should be determined as the interventions are developed. The interventions should clearly state the key changes that address the contributing factors identified in the in-depth analysis of the event. To avoid frustration and to fight the urge to create the perfect plan, the action plan should represent small tests of change. The

Plan-Do-Study-Act (PDSA) model, a rapid cycle of process improvement, has been used in a number of safety projects (see Chapter 7).

Another suggestion in planning and implementing a safety project is for the group to network with internal and external resources when developing strategies. Internal resources may include new group members from information systems, or other units who are working on the same or similar problems or projects. External organizations such as The Agency for Healthcare Research and Quality (AHRQ), the Institute for Healthcare Improvement (IHI), and the Joint Commission on Accreditation of Healthcare Organizations (JCAHO) are just a few of the agencies that can provide information on evidence-based safety practices and protocols. (See Chapter 10 for further information on internal and external resources.)

The specific implementation plan will need to be developed by the team based on the problem and the contributing factors. However, the following suggestions may be helpful in addressing some of the more frequent contributing factors.

Many tasks can be improved through standardization and built-in double-check systems. The use of protocols and checklists may help with many of the routine tasks and procedures used in patient care. These tools can help reduce the risk of forgetting key steps and educating those who may be unfamiliar with the process. Checklists can help to build redundant checks of key interventions by various disciplines and increase the certainty that essential tasks are completed (Piotrowski & Hinshaw, 2002). This is especially helpful where role overlap can occur. The use of protocols should be viewed as suggestions for care, and the contraindications for their use should be included where appropriate (Maddox, Wakefield, & Bull, 2001).

The myriad of problems attributed to team functioning can often be addressed through efforts to improve communication, both written and verbal. For example, the strategy of a daily goals and objectives sheet has been instrumental in improving the communication of the plan of care in the ICU setting (Pronovost et al., 2003). The sheet, developed through the collaborative effort of the team members of an academic 16-bed surgical oncology ICU, serves as an interdisciplinary communication tool and checklist for the daily plan for each patient. The goals are clearly stated along with the plan for any tests or procedures, and safety precautions or protocols that should be observed (Johns Hopkins University School of Medicine, 2002). The attention given to the completion of an interdisciplinary tool reinforces that safety is more than a project; it is a shared value of the team.

Working conditions and individual provider factors can be optimized by giving greater attention to the material and human resources that support the immediate environment for patient care. Shortcuts or work-arounds are less likely when staff are provided with supplies and equipment that are readily available and in good working order. Distractions and injuries are fewer with ample space, adequate lighting, and less noise in the environment. Factors such as shift length, shift rotation, and staffing ratios should be evaluated for their potential contribution to fatigue and stress (Maddox, Wakefield, & Bull, 2001).

The IOM (2001) report, *Crossing the Quality Chasm: A New Health System for the 21st Century,* notes the use of information technology as one of the first critical steps in transforming the healthcare delivery system and improving safety and quality. Technological supports, such as computerized order entry and automated systems that include decision support and safety rules, can address a number of factors that contribute to error. Clinicians need to fully understand the process of care and possible contributing factors for error in order to select the correct technological features and to use them safely.

Steps 6 and 7: Document the Results and Share the Stories

The progress of the project should be *visible* to the team members. Frequent feedback will be a key factor in the success of the project. Again, the use of data and concrete information will reinforce to the team that safety is not improved by blame and ridicule but by achieving a change in the system. Rapid turnaround of the results not only lets the team know their progress, but also helps them to *feel* supported in their effort (Piotrowski & Hinshaw, 2002). The feedback further allows the team to make the necessary mid-course corrections if a particular strategy or set of strategies is not working. Documentation of the results and sharing the stories helps others to *hear* about the progress and the obstacles or barriers encountered. Presenting a balanced picture of the effort will help to spread improvements to other areas and keep the problem spots on the radar screen for the organization.

Step 8: Resurvey Staff

The initial safety climate survey should be repeated following the implementation of changes, and periodically thereafter. The perceptions or *feelings* of the team should be reassessed to determine if the culture has shifted toward one that values safety as a priority. It is unlikely that a sweeping change will occur with just one effort, and the gradual shift may need to be monitored over time. The team may discover that additional disciplines need to be included more actively in projects to create a change in culture. Leadership can use these results to target support to foster the evolution of a culture of safety.

Role of the Nurse in Planning a Safety Project

Although many disciplines are involved in the overall plan of care, nurses are major drivers of performance improvement activities. Out of all the care team members, it is the nurse who remains in the closest proximity to the patient around the clock. Throughout the education and professional training of nurses, our duty as a patient advocate is reinforced. As such, we typically, and quite capably, fix things. We fix what is late, inadequate, or flat out wrong or unsafe. We can easily identify what is wrong, but need to become more adept at helping to identify how things can be fixed to make, and keep, them working correctly. Nurses can be influential in shaping the agenda for improving safety through their role in planning safety projects. Key aspects of the role that deserve attention are creating the vision for safety, fostering collaboration and relationship-centered health care with other disciplines, and developing data competency and analytical skills (see Table 3.3).

Table 3.3   Role of the Nurse in Safety Projects

Role Aspect	Exemplars
Creating the vision	Keep projects "patient-focused." Strive to elevate goals. Advocate for evidence-based, best practices.
Fostering collaboration	Employ active listening skills. Encourage shared decision making. Demonstrate respect and empathy.
Data competency and analytical skills	Use data as objective evidence. Gather and give the appropriate facts.

Making the Vision a Reality

Nurses play a vital role in shaping the future for patient safety because they are so involved in the implementation of safe processes and are "patient-focused." They possess first-hand knowledge of the complexity of everyday problems that can be crafted into many mini-projects as part of an overall plan to improve the level of care. Each initiative should drive toward the common goal of improving the safety of the environment for patients and the staff.

As an active participant in the process to make the vision of a safe environment a reality, nurses should strive to use their influence to achieve outcomes that rise above mediocrity. Practice changes that improve safety represent best practices, and by monitoring outcomes nurses can provide the evidence needed for evidence-based decision making.

Fostering Collaboration and Patient-Centered Health Care

Traditional models of education and professional training foster the development of a discipline-specific focus on patient care. However, as the acuity of hospitalized patients has grown, so has the interdependence of the various healthcare disciplines. The complexity of many of the safety issues illustrates that no single discipline has all the information, skills, or resources to solve the problem. Nurses will need to become comfortable sharing the work and developing expertise as a collaborative team member. Collaboration and relationship-centered care that is based on active listening, shared decision making, trust, empathy, and respect form the basis for the partnership that is necessary to improve the quality and safety of patient care (Sherwood, Thomas, Bennett, & Lewis, 2002). Encouraging a partnership with the patient and family to ensure safety will be largely dependent on the collaboration and effectiveness of the healthcare team.

Competency in Data Management and Analytical Skills

Given the strong intuitive sense that many nurses have, there is a tendency to rely on gut feelings and to speak in general terms. Proving your point through the use of objective data is necessary to solicit the support of other healthcare team members and to convince them of the progress along the way. Data competency is more than manipulating numbers in a spreadsheet. Turning data into information that can be used to make decisions includes a process in which the team asks the right questions; collects and analyzes the data in an appropriate and usable form; provides critical information; displays the data in a usable, interpretable way; disseminates the importance of the problem; and monitors results (Newhouse & Mills, 2002). Competency in the management of data will be critical to secure collaboration with multi-disciplinary team members and communicate to and solicit support from administration.

Conclusion

Nurses make up the largest portion of the healthcare workforce and can play a powerful role in creating an environment of safety. A comprehensive safety program can transcend the focus of fixing a single problem, creating a change in the way the healthcare team thinks about and responds to safety concerns. The nurse can facilitate the interdisciplinary process by using the eight-step method to help the team get a feel for the culture related to safety, hear more about the science of safety, sniff out opportunities to improve safety, take a critical look at the system and care processes, create a shared vision and effort for improving care, see the changes that are made, and determine whether the change improves the safety of patients. In order to fuel the momentum of change for the team, the nurse needs to create the vision for patient safety, foster the collaboration of the team, and assist with or lead in the review and analysis of the data so that improvements can result.

References

Bower, J. O. (2002). Designing and implementing a patient safety program for the OR. *Association of Operating Room Nurses, 76*(3), 452–456.

Feinstein, K. W., Grunden, N., & Harrison, E. I. (2002). A region addresses patient safety. *American Journal of Infection Control, 30*(4), 248–251.

Institute of Medicine. (2001). *Crossing the quality chasm: A new health system for the 21st century.* Washington, DC: National Academy Press.

Johns Hopkins University School of Medicine. (2002). *Making a science of patient safety: A systematic, eight-step quality process in surgical ICUs.* Retrieved April 24, 2003, from Institute for Healthcare Improvement web site: http://www.ihi.org/newsandpublications/other/ICU.pdf

Ketring, S. P., & White, J. P. (2002). Developing a systemwide approach to patient safety: The first year. *The Joint Commission Journal on Quality Improvement, 28*(6), 287–295.

Maddox, P. J., Wakefield, M., & Bull, J. (2001). Patient safety and the need for professional and educational change. *Nursing Outlook, 49*(1), 8–13.

Mawji, Z., Stillman, P., Laskowski, R., Lawrence, S., Karoly, E., Capuano, T., & Sussman, E. (2002). First do no harm: Integrating patient safety and quality improvement. *The Joint Commission Journal on Quality Improvement, 28*(7), 373–386.

Newhouse, R. P. & Mills, M. E. (2002). *Nursing leadership in the acute care setting of the organized delivery system.* Washington, DC: ANA-Publishing.

Piotrowski, M. M., & Hinshaw, D. B. (2002). The safety checklist program: Creating a culture of safety in intensive care units. *The Joint Commission Journal on Quality Improvement, 28*(6), 306–315.

Pronovost, P., Berenholtz, S., Dorman, T., Lipsett, P. A., Simmonds, T., & Haraden, C. (2003). Improving communication in the ICU using daily goals. *Journal of Critical Care, 18*(2), 71–75.

Pronovost, P., Wu., A. W., Dorman, T., & Morlock, L. (2002). Building safety into ICU care. *Journal of Critical Care, 17*(2), 78–85.

Sexton, B. J., Helmreich, R., Pronovost, P. J., & Thomas, E. (2003). *Safety climate survey.* Retrieved September 25, 2003, from Institute for Healthcare Improvement web site: http://www.qualityhealthcare.org/NR/rdonlyres/145C0998-5FB4-46EA-8CFD-D08D3CE9082C/797/SafetyClimateSurvey.pdf

Sherwood, G., Thomas, E., Bennett, D. S., & Lewis, P. (2002). A teamwork model to promote patient safety in critical care. *Critical Care Clinics of North America, 14,* 333–340.

Shojania, K. G., Wald, H., & Gross, R. (2002). Understanding medical error and improving patient safety in the inpatient setting. *Medical Clinics of North America, 86*(4), 847–867.

The University of Texas at Austin. (2002). *Safety attitudes questionnaire.*

Wong, P., Helsinger, D., & Petry, J. (2002). Providing the right infrastructure to lead the culture change for patient safety. *The Joint Commission Journal on Quality Improvement, 28*(7), 363–372.

CHAPTER 4

Rapid Cycle Safety Improvement

Terry Nelson, MSN, RN, Assistant Director, Medical Nursing Service*
Stephanie S. Poe, MScN, RN, Coordinator for Nursing Clinical Quality*

On reviewing the latest medication event trends for the medical intensive care unit (MICU), members of the Performance Improvement (PI) committee notice that far too many medication errors are resulting from using intravenous (IV) infusion pumps to deliver sedation boluses. These errors appear to follow a similar pattern: A critically ill patient needs sedation to prevent self-injury; a nurse administers the sedation bolus by increasing the IV pump rate to a high rate; the nurse then forgets to reset the IV pump at the prescribed lower rate after the bolus is completed. Despite staff reminders that greater attention to safety is needed when giving IV boluses, errors of this nature persist. Although no patient has been harmed to date, you and your colleagues feel that you need to improve the safety of sedation boluses as soon as possible.

The Joint Commission on Accreditation of Healthcare Organizations (JCAHO) encourages integration of safety priorities into the design and redesign of all relevant organizational processes, functions, and services as part of improving organizational performance (JCAHO, 2002). Once the decision is made to improve the quality and safety of the healthcare system, teams need to select a method for improvement. A variety of quality and performance improvement (PI) tools and methodologies are available from which to choose. Which methodology to use is generally determined at the organizational level, so that a consistent approach is applied to all PI activities, including those designed to reduce safety risks. Due to time and resource constraints, rapid cycle methodologies are becoming increasing popular.

*The Johns Hopkins Hospital

The overall aim of this chapter is to provide clinical nurse leaders, educators, and managers with a toolbox for rapid cycle change. The objectives of this chapter are to:

- Describe current quality improvement methods
- Describe the Model for Improvement
- Identify critical questions to answer before embarking on change
- Describe how to use PDSA cycles for testing changes
- Describe how the Model for Improvement was used to enhance medication safety in a medical intensive care unit

Current Quality Improvement Methods

According to Benedetto (2003), PI methods can be grouped into two broad categories—revolutionary methods and evolutionary methods. Revolutionary methods such as re-engineering and Six Sigma are labor and resource intensive and are best reserved for times when major process redesign is needed. Six Sigma, which is a system-wide data-driven business strategy, focuses on eliminating defects or errors, identifying sources of variation and opportunities for standardization, and applying controls to maintain the improvements (Lanham & Maxson-Cooper, 2003). The model includes the five phases summarized by the acronym DMAIC: define, measure, analyze, improve, and control.

Evolutionary improvement methods such as quality circles, continuous quality improvement, and total quality management work well when small incremental improvements are desired, when significant process redesign is not needed, and when the avoidance of disruption of work flow is desired (Benedetto, 2003). Today's healthcare system is in continual flux, and many organizations are reluctant to make drastic and radical changes that could significantly affect operations and work flow. For this reason, evolutionary models such as the Model for Improvement, originally described by Langley, Nolan, and Nolan (1992), are gaining popularity (Figure 4.1). These models incorporate the concepts of rapid cycle change and measurement for learning. The JCAHO uses a similar cycle for improving performance, which directs teams to systematically and scientifically design, collect data, aggregate and analyze data, improve, and redesign/design (JCAHO, 2000).

The Model for Improvement

The Johns Hopkins Hospital uses the Model for Improvement to guide many of its PI and safety improvement efforts. This evolutionary model was selected because of its simplicity and its effectiveness in producing change with minimal interruption in workflow. The model includes a reflective component and

Figure 4.1   The Model for Improvement

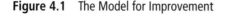

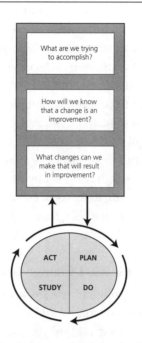

Source: The Improvement Guide. A Practical Approach to Enhancing Organizational Performance. Langley, Nolan, Nolan, Norman, & Provost. Copyright (c) 1996 by Gerald J. Langley, Kevin M. Nolan, Thomas W. Nolan, Clifford L. Norman, & Lloyd P. Provost. Reprinted by permission of John Wiley & Sons, Inc.

an active component and attempts to analyze and improve processes by initially testing change on a small scale prior to wide dissemination (Berwick, 1996). During reflection, teams strive to identify goals, metrics, and change strategies by asking themselves: What is our goal? How will we know when we reach our goal? What changes will we make to achieve our goal? Once these questions have been answered, the team actively uses learning cycles to plan and test changes in systems and processes. These learning cycles, usually referred to as Plan-Do-Study-Act (PDSA) cycles, were originally described by Shewhart (1931).

Reflection: The Critical Questions

What Are We Trying to Accomplish?

Before you can embark on a safety improvement project, you need to decide what it is that you are trying to accomplish. System change requires will, and one way that the will for improvement can be translated is to set aims that clearly articulate the level of system performance required (Nolan, 2000). Teams must have the desire to improve. Lasting improvement is not an accident, but rather comes from committed people who have a clear idea of what they want to accomplish. A clear, well-defined aim with a defined numerical goal increases the likelihood of improvement.

Assembling a team of people committed to a common goal is essential to accomplishing that goal. Ideal team members are people who know the process well, line managers, financial and data support resources, stakeholders, and individuals with sufficient authority in the organization to help recognize and move systems barriers. It is useful to select individuals of various skills and personalities. For example, the team should contain both creative individuals and those who will concentrate on project completion. Individuals of various disciplines should be included as team members because of their varying knowledge of the process and insight into improvement options. Many patient safety initiatives require the cooperation and leadership of physicians. When physicians are key drivers of the process, having a physician champion is a definite plus. These powerful supporters are in the best position to convince their colleagues that the changes identified are feasible, safe, and advantageous (Institute of Healthcare Improvement, 2003).

How Will We Know That Change Is an Improvement?

Once you have a committed team dedicated to accomplishing a well-defined aim, you need to determine what would constitute an improvement. In order to do this, you need to understand how the process works and how it currently varies.

At the start of a safety improvement process, flowcharting is a useful technique to help you understand how the process of interest currently works. Software packages such as Microsoft Visio Professional 2002 simplify the construction of flowcharts. The flowchart, or flow diagram, uses graphic symbols to depict the nature and flow of the steps in a process from beginning to end (iSixSigma, 2000). The process can be mapped out at a high level (major steps) or at a more granular (detailed) level, and uses symbols that are common across industries (Figure 4.2). These symbols identify points at which decisions are made, delays occur, and reports are produced. Breaking the process down into steps allows team members to identify problem areas and provides opportunities for simplification or elim-

Figure 4.2   Common Flow Chart Symbols

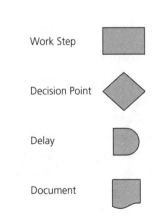

ination of redundancies. Front-line individuals who use the process on a day-to-day basis often most accurately provide content for the flowchart and are in the best position to identify problem areas. Although overall agreement by the workgroup on the accuracy of the process depicted by the flowchart is important, you should avoid spending excessive time striving for perfection, because this can delay progress.

Once the process is understood, the team needs to establish simple measures that will show if a change leads to an improvement. Berwick (1996) pictures measurement as a handmaiden to improvement, stating that improvement cannot act without it. Measurement for the purposes of learning helps us to clarify our aim and to know whether a selected change should be maintained, revised, or tossed out.

Depending upon the project aim, safety improvement measures can address a need to learn more about the clinical, service, fiscal, or infrastructure aspects of care that affect patient safety. Measures with a clinical focus can include nosocomial infection rates, fall injury rates, and medication error rates. Service measures, also important to health care as a service industry, can include the number of patient complaints, customer and employee satisfaction scores, and internal interdepartmental satisfaction scores. Fiscal measures can include length of hospital stay, denied inpatient hospital days, case mix intensity, collection rate, and charge per case. Finally, infrastructure measures gauge the effectiveness of key points of the infrastructure, such as time until new outpatient appointment, emergency department walk-out rates, and percentage of times when operating room cases start on time. Chapter 5 describes measurement in further detail.

What Changes Can We Make that Will Result in Improvement?

When you look at the process of interest, do you envision particular ideas for improvement? Can needless complexity or redundancy be eliminated? Is there consensus on the best way for this process to work? It is important to "think outside the box" at this juncture. New results cannot come from old methods. Langley and colleagues (1996) have outlined six guiding principles for creative thinking: challenge the boundaries, rearrange the order of steps, look for ways to smooth the flow of activities, evaluate the purpose, visualize the ideal, and remove "the current way of doing things" as an option. Brainstorm a variety of actions that could potentially result in an improved process. Then, after team discussion, prioritize the list and select one small change to pilot test first.

Action

Once the reflective component is completed, the safety improvement team actively uses rapid learning cycles to plan and test changes in systems and processes. This PDSA approach, based on work by W. Edwards Deming for testing and quality improvement and developed by Shewhart (1931), is easy to understand, provides quick results, has been tested in a variety of settings, and is applicable for both clinical and nonclinical areas. Additionally, the model is a scientific method, encourages measurement, and is broadly supported in the literature. The cycle begins with the development of a plan and ends with actions based on the knowledge acquired during the Plan, Do, and Study phases of the cycle (Langley et al., 1996). Table 4.1 outlines steps in the PDSA cycle. Additional cycles are used to refine or monitor the initial change or to test other changes.

Table 4.1   Steps in the Plan-Do-Study-Act (PDSA) Model

Step	Definition
Plan	State improvement goal, predict outcome, and develop strategy to test change.
Do	Implement a small change. Document lessons learned and begin data analysis.
Study	Complete data analysis, identify lessons learned, and display results.
Act	Communicate results. Build successful change into current processes. Analyze failures for change opportunities. Plan for next change to test.

Plan

All effective action begins with a plan. During the *plan* phase, the details of the pilot test of change are outlined and predictions as to the outcomes of the change are put forward. The goal of the pilot test should be clearly stated and documented. Next, team members should predict the outcome of the selected change. A detailed plan follows, and should include the answers to the "who-what-when-where-how" questions.

Who will test the change and who will collect and analyze the data? What change will be made and what specific data will be necessary to collect? When will the change be tested and when will data collection and analysis begin and end? Where will the change be tested and from where will the data be derived? How will the change be tested and how will data be collected, analyzed, and communicated?

The data collection and analysis plan is an important component of the planning process. Data may be collected from existing databases, reports, surveys, or observational sources. The source must be a reliable one that will be available in the future to help provide further data. Additionally, external benchmarks may be useful so that the process can be compared with others outside the organization.

A team member with specific competencies in data management, analysis, and reporting needs to be identified during the planning phase. You may need to hire an outside consultant if the team does not include someone who possesses these skills. What software package will be used? Does that individual have the necessary hardware and software to accomplish the task? How will the team want to display data? Will bar graphs, line graphs, pie charts, run charts, or other types of displays be generated? Once the plan has been developed, you are ready to move on to the next phase of the cycle.

Table 4.3 Possible Contributors to Unsuccessful Change

Inadequate skill, knowledge, or training
Ineffective job aids
Inappropriate workload
Inadequate assistance from personnel or technology
Inadequate work conditions
Inefficient work design
Inadequate performance feedback
Unpleasant or punitive task
Task or role confusion
Consequences do not support performance desired

Case Study

What Were We Trying to Accomplish?

- *Motivation:* Four potentially serious medication events involving IV sedation bolus administration were reported over a 2-year period.

- *Aim:* To improve the safety of IV sedation bolus administration.

- *Team members:* A clinical nurse specialist (leader and facilitator); a pharmacist clinical specialist; nurse representatives from intensive care units across the hospital; a nurse educator; the Associate Director of Health, Epidemiology, and Infection Control, who acted as a resource person to the group; an IV pump vendor representative; and an intensivist (physician champion).

How Would We Know That Change Was an Improvement?

- *Current process:* MICU staff routinely administer frequent sedation in order to provide adequate pain relief and comfort during mechanical ventilation and bedside procedures. Sedation is typically administered with a bolus from a pharmacy-mixed IV solution of fentanyl or midazolam. Such boluses typically have been administered by reprogramming the infusion pump to run at 999 mL/hour for several minutes, returning to the original rate after the bolus amount has infused. Despite attention to patient safety and a high nurse-to-patient ratio, the ICU nurse is subjected to frequent interruptions and distractions. Although the pump alarms upon bolus completion, the potential for delay or error in pump reprogramming is high.

■ *Measures:* Number of self-reported actual or potential IV sedation errors and nurse satisfaction with the changed process.

What Changes Could We Make That Would Result in Improvement?

■ *Proposed changes:* A variety of changes were proposed to replace the dose calculation method for IV boluses and adapt the safest available procedure(s) in MICU; explore testing of new technology that incorporates safety features that either prevent or mitigate harm to patients.

■ *Selected change to pilot test:* IV pump equipped with "smart-pump" technology that can be preprogrammed to allow the pump to reset itself after the bolus is administered and has programmable and nonprogrammable limits as safety features.

PDSA

■ *Plan:* A plan was developed for MICU nurses to pilot the "smart-pump" technology in all MICU patients for a 30-day period in November 2002. This plan included a detailed methodology for obtaining data from the internal pump data management system and the institution's online medication event system, as well as a tool for measuring nurse satisfaction data.

■ *Do:* During initial testing of the process change, there were two sedation bolus events. The test pump did not allow the nurse to view the dose scrolling across the IV pump screen, nor did it allow the nurse to use a dose key to enable the pump to calculate the rate based on a nurse-entered dose. Not having a visible dose scrolling across the pump was a factor in both errors. Because nurses would no longer be able to visualize a scrolling dose, MICU instituted preprinted labels to enable easy identification of the drug doses and the pump channel containing these drugs. In addition, the pilot was delayed due to contract issues and the need for corporate purchasing involvement.

■ *Study:* During the pilot, the pump's internal settings alerted staff to 70 potential events in which human programming errors would have resulted in either a low rate or potentially dangerous rate for the patient. For example, a heparin infusion was initially programmed to infuse at 10,000 units/hour. The hard "guardrail," which was set for 300 units/hr, alerted the user of the programming error, and the infusion was reprogrammed to the prescribed rate. Analysis of nurse satisfaction data revealed that over 96 percent of nurses participating in the pilot felt safer using the trial pump.

■ *Act:* Communication of pilot results was widespread, and hospital stakeholders were impressed with the safety features of the new pumps. Taking into account vendor contract timing and budgetary considerations, clinical and financial leadership approved initial funding for IV pump replacements in high risk areas, such as intensive care, intermediate care, post-anesthesia care, and operating room areas. The long-term plan is to replace the remaining fleet over time.

Conclusion

The immediacy of the desire to make a change once a risk area has been identified is part of human nature. No one consciously wants to continue to perform in an unsafe practice environment. This violates the primary directive of healthcare team members to "do no harm." For this reason, healthcare teams find that, if they do not like the current level of patient safety afforded by their system, they must change the institutional risk profile by improving that system. Furthermore, they recognize that they need to do so in the best time- and resource-efficient manner, given competing patient care priorities. The application of the concepts of rapid cycle change and measurement for learning as described in this chapter enables teams to test and implement changes in a structured and reflective manner. Nurse leaders play a critical role in instituting PI methodologies that improve the quality and safety of patient care with minimal disruption of day-to-day operations.

References

Benedetto, A. R. (2003). Six Sigma: Not for the faint of heart. *Radiology Management, 25*(2), 40–53.

Berwick, D. (1996). A primer on leading the improvement of systems. *British Medical Journal, 312,* 619–622.

Institute of Healthcare Improvement. (2003). IHI quality improvement resources: A model for accelerating improvement. Retrieved August 29, 2003, from http://www.ihi.org/resources/qi

iSixSigma. (2000). Process mapping and flow charting. Retrieved August 29, 2003, from http://www.isixsigma.com

Joint Commission on Accreditation of Healthcare Organizations (2000). Advanced performance improvement for hospitals. JCAHO: Oakbrook Terrace: IL.

Joint Commission Resources (2002). Sentinel event alert advisory group identifies JCAHO's 2003 national patient safety goals. *Joint Commission Perspectives on Patient Safety, 2*(9), 1, 3.

Langley, G. L., Nolan, K. M., Nolan, T. W. (1992). *The foundation of improvement.* Silver Spring, MD: API.

Langley, G. L., Nolan, K. M., Nolan, T. W., Norman, C. L., & Provost, L. P. (1996). *The improvement guide: A practical approach to enhancing organizational performance.* San Francisco, CA: Jossey-Bass.

Lanham, B., & Maxson-Cooper, P. (2003). Is Six Sigma the answer for nursing to reduce medical errors and enhance patient safety? *Nursing Economic$, 21*(1), 39–41, 38.

Nolan, T. W. (2000). System changes to improve patient safety. *British Medical Journal, 320,* 771–773.

Shewhart, W. A. (1931). *Economic control of quality of manufactured product.* New York: Van Nostrand. (Reprinted Milwaukee, WI: American Society for Quality Control, 1980.)

CHAPTER 5

The Metrics of Measuring Patient Safety

Robin P. Newhouse, RN, Ph.D.
Nurse Researcher/Assistant Professor*

I t was going to be a busy day. It was 7 AM, and an emergency was on its way to the OR. The perioperative nurse prepared the instruments and equipment and completed the preoperative assessment. The patient was rolled into the room, and when the nurse reached for the safety strap that secures the patient on the bed, it was missing. She had checked her room to ensure that all equipment was available prior to the start of her first case, but in the emergent situation, had missed the safety strap. This was the second time that this had happened. She informed the charge nurse that equipment was missing, and found another safety strap. The perioperative nurse discussed the problem with the charge nurse, and with a team of peers developed a standard room checklist that could be used. Equipment availability improved, and a system was put into place that decreases the chance of a patient fall.

In this situation, the perioperative nurse identified a problem and achieved a short-term resolution. To make an impact on error reduction, a system approach, detailing specific aims and measurements, is required (Berwick, 1996). This system approach will be realized through collaborative efforts. For these collaborative efforts to be successful, the nurse's participation and leadership are essential.

Nurses are fundamental to the healthcare improvement team because they are intimately involved in the processes of care and contribute uniquely to the safe environment for patients. Nurses contribute to and lead

*The Johns Hopkins Hospital/The Johns Hopkins University School of Nursing

performance improvement teams that are responsible for developing measures, collecting primary data, analyzing that data, and making changes based on that data to improve care for patients. Appropriate measures must be used to capture these improvements and communicate valid suggestions to the team who will make the process changes. Establishing the need for change with the healthcare team is critical for the implementation of practice changes.

In addition to understanding the need for change, using strong measurement allows teams to articulate the impact of improvements to their unit, organizationally, or externally to professional or policy audiences. Measurement will lead to improvements in care, but measurement requires that the purpose of the measure is clear, the goals of the measure are focused, and the validity and reliability of the measure are established (Berwick, James, & Coye, 2003). Skill in measurement and interpretation of outcomes are essential for nurse leaders involved in safety initiatives and will serve them well, building their professional credibility and value to the team.

To measure safety improvements, nurse leaders will need to choose a significant problem, implement a strategy to improve safety, and use a measure that is appropriate for the problem. To build these skills, this chapter will cover issues related to the measurement component of measuring patient safety. The objectives of this chapter are to:

- Describe the process for selecting a patient safety measure
- Identify patient safety measures of structure, process, and outcome

Selecting a Patient Safety Measure

Table 5.1 provides some common definitions for the concepts of measurement, safety, outcomes, and measure used in this chapter. A patient safety measure refers to an instrument by which phenomena (structures, processes, or outcomes) related to patient safety are quantified or translated into numbers. This conversion to numbers allows healthcare teams to translate data into information, so that the clinical implications of the data can be assessed and acted upon to improve patient care. Selecting a patient safety measure requires a systematic approach. We need a measure, or quantity, to understand the effect of our care and the impact of our improvements. We cannot improve what we cannot measure, so the measure is a pivotal aspect of any improvement effort.

This approach involves assuring that the problem is clearly identified and refined, possible options are reviewed, and the measure is selected based on its ability to capture the phenomena of interest (validity) in a reproducible manner (reliability). The patient safety measure will need to withstand the team's evaluation and pilot testing. The first step is to identify the problem.

Table 5.1   Concept Definitions

Concept	Definition and Source
Measurement	The assignment of numbers to objects according to specified rules to characterize quantities of an attribute. (Polit & Beck, 2004)
Safety	Freedom from accidental injury. (Committee on Quality of Health Care in America, 1999)
Outcomes	Favorable or adverse changes in the actual or potential health status of persons, groups, or communities that can be attributed to prior or concurrent care. (Donabedian, 1985, p. 256)
Measure or Instrument	A device and method by which characteristics or phenomena (structures, processes, or outcomes) of interest are quantified, or translated into numbers. (Waltz, Strickland, & Lenz, 1991)

Identifying the Problem to Be Measured

Patient safety problems emerge from multiple sources. They may arise in clinical experience (e.g., performance improvement, staff meetings, close calls, sentinel events), communication from external regulatory agencies (e.g., quality measures of the Joint Commission or Sentinel Event Alerts) or professional sources (e.g., professional journal, standards, or networking at conferences), or from patients' feedback. Other times the problem may be presented by public media such as newspapers (Berens, 2002) or research reports (Miller et al., 2001; Miller, Elixhauser, & Zhan, 2003). It is also useful to list common published patient safety problems, asking nurses to rate to what extent each issue exists on their unit. This strategy will provide means (averages) and a hierarchy to prioritize discussion with unit staff to probe the issues. An example based on commonly identified safety problems by Kinzer (2001) can be viewed in Table 5.2.

When the problem is identified, the Plan-Do-Study-Act (PDSA) process can be used to frame the safety action plans (see Chapter 4). The next step is to choose a measure so that baseline data can be collected to determine or validate the extent of the problem, and provide the starting point for the performance improvement effort. This measure is the concept of interest described in a quantifiable definition reduced to numbers or categories, also known as a metric or indicator. Pronovost et al. (2001) suggest a process of developing a quality measure. This process includes selecting, designing, and evaluating the measure. In this chapter, we will limit the discussion to the component of quality that relates to patient safety.

Table 5.2 Example of Questions to Identify Unit Safety Problems

Check the response that most closely represents your answer to this question: To what extent do these issues exist in our unit?			
To what extent do these issues exist on our unit?	To no extent (0)	To some extent (1)	To a great extent (2)
Being time-pressured	❏	❏	❏
Many different types of equipment	❏	❏	❏
Multiple individuals involved in the care of individual patients	❏	❏	❏
High volume and/or unpredictable patient flow	❏	❏	❏
Need for rapid care management decisions	❏	❏	❏
Communication problems with co-workers	❏	❏	❏
Multiple "hand offs" in care	❏	❏	❏
Environment distractions	❏	❏	❏
High acuity of patient illness or injury	❏	❏	❏
Inexperienced caregivers	❏	❏	❏
Diagnostic or therapeutic interventions having a narrow margin of safety	❏	❏	❏
Communication barriers with patients	❏	❏	❏

Source: Adapted from Kinzer (2001).

Team Decisions

When approaching the measurement of a safety concept, one of the major challenges is choosing the measure. The team will be faced with finding an established measure, adapting a measure to meet their needs, or creating their own measure. After the concept is refined to reflect the problem, the best choice is to find an existing measure. The first reason for this choice is that your team can then benchmark (compare) progress against other organizations or units with similar problems. The second reason is that established measures may have reliability (consistent and stable scores) and validity (represents the concept of interest) estimated, adding to the confidence in your results and recommendations. If the measure is not publicly available, then the team may need to request permission from the author to use the instrument. If you need to adapt or create a measure, then it may be useful for your improvement effort, but you will lose the ability to benchmark results against similar settings.

When approaching measure selection for Performance Improvement (PI), you should establish a set of criteria. The Strategic Framework Board of the National Quality Measurement and Reporting System has published four hierarchical criteria sets for evaluating national quality measures: importance, scientific acceptability, usability, and feasibility (McGlynn, 2003). To get the most benefit from the measure selection process, data needed to determine performance must be readily available and accessible to clinicians within the flow of their work. These principles hold true for local performance measures as well. Interdisciplinary safety-focused PI teams should learn to choose measures that have clinical or practical meaning; are useful for decision making regarding goal-directed change; and are reliable, valid, adaptable, and feasible to implement.

Pronovost and Berenholtz (2002) outline six steps to select and develop quality measures in the intensive care unit (ICU) environment, which were adopted from McGlynn (1998): conducting a systematic literature review, selecting specific types of outcomes to evaluate, selecting pilot measures, writing design specifications for the measures, evaluating the validity and reliability of the data, and pilot testing the measures. To keep the team on track, target dates for completing each task and responsibility should be assigned (see Table 5.3).

Table 5.3 Projecting the Timing for Developing a Patient Safety Measure

Steps	Target Date	Responsibility
1. Conducting a systematic literature review		
2. Selecting specific types of outcomes to evaluate		
3. Selecting pilot measures		
4. Writing design specifications for the measures		
5. Evaluating the validity and reliability of the data		
6. Pilot testing the measures		

Interdisciplinary, safety-focused PI teams in ICUs would find Pronovost and Berenholtz's (2002; 2004) monographs of great value as they present quality indicators developed specifically for the ICU environment, as well as the evidence supporting their selection.

Conducting a Systematic Literature Review

The first step is to conduct a literature review to determine what reported data exist, the reported links between processes and outcomes, and the instruments that were used. Resources accessed should include a range of sources, such as print and electronic resources, professional organizations, regulatory sources, and non-profit organizations. This will give the team a working knowledge of the content area of interest. (See Chapter 11 for a compilation of publicly available resources.)

Selecting Specific Types of Outcomes to Evaluate

Next, the team must determine what outcome is important. This will drive the selection of structures and processes chosen for study and subsequent improvements. Patient safety measures focus on structures and processes that are associated with patient injury or adverse health. Specific examples of structures, processes, and outcome measures will be explained further later in this chapter.

If the team cannot find any established measures in the literature review, they will need to construct their own by defining the concept of interest, constructing observable indicators, developing the measure, and then evaluating the measure through pilot testing (Waltz, Strickland, & Lenz, 1991). Consulting an expert on metrics or using a reference to guide the team is recommended (Pronovost & Moen, 2003).

Selecting Pilot Measures

In selecting the pilot measures, the team will need to determine the type of measure, evaluate the strength of evidence supporting the use of the measure, and evaluate the feasibility of data collection (Pronovost et al., 2001). The evidence supporting the use of the measure is the reliability and validity of the measure, and the scope of the measure's use within and outside the organization documented in your literature and resource review (step one). The measure must also have practical utility to clinicians and be feasible to administer; in other words, the burden of data collection, or time required, should be acceptable and attainable for the clinical staff. They should also be user interpretable, so that there is no error when the measures are utilized. Test the measure in a small pilot sample to validate that it is appropriate for your project.

The data collection and plan also need to consider the ethical implications of data collection; for example, if there are concerns about the effect of a new product on the nosocomial infection rate for central lines, it would be harmful to patients to test the product to determine the infection rate. A second ethical consideration is to be clear about the goal of data collection. Data collected specifically to understand a process or customers, or to evaluate changes, that is focused on the improvement of care for patients is usually considered performance improvement (Solberg, Mosser, & McDonald, 1997). Data collected to generate knowledge beyond what is required for clinical performance improvement is considered research (Solberg et al., 1997). Once the purpose has shifted to research, or if the intent of the team is to publish results, Institutional Review Board approval must be obtained prior to starting the project to assure compliance with human subject protection as well as the patients' rights to privacy in light of recent Health Insurance Portability and Accountability Act (HIPAA) regulations.

Writing Design Specifications for the Measures

Writing design specifications includes defining the details of data collection, including responsibility, timing, setting, and methods (instruments and technology). It also involves selecting a unit of analysis, defining the indicator, identifying the target population, defining the risk adjustment strategy, and identifying the data sources (Pronovost et al., 2001).

First, selecting the unit of analysis involves deciding if the patient safety measure will represent the patient level, the unit level, or the organizational level. If you are engaged in a PI effort (discussed in Chapter 2), you will most likely be collecting data at the patient level and reporting it at the unit level. Other projects may focus on a specific patient population on the unit, or a population that transcends units or the organization. For example, for patients discharged after an admission with a diagnosis of congestive heart failure or community-acquired pneumonia, the team may focus on compliance with smoking cessation education prior to discharge. Percentages of compliance with smoking cessation can be reported by organization or by unit. This type of data may also be reported at the organizational level through external quality indicator projects such as The Quality Indicator Project by The Association of Maryland Hospitals & Health Systems (2003).

Next, consider if a risk adjustment strategy is needed. Risk adjustment is a mechanism to improve comparisons between findings, so that the results are comparable, or the patients in the sample are similar. Similar patients can be chosen for the sample, or there should be some way to stratify the co-morbidities (other illnesses) and severity (how sick the patient is). For example, if you are reviewing cardiac surgery outcomes, you may want to risk adjust by either using similar patients or adjusting by diagnosis, surgery time, and American Society of Anesthesiologists (ASA) score. The ASA score is a measure of anesthesia risk (American Society of Anesthesiologists, 2003). Risk adjusting will help the team to interpret the data and to explain if the outcome is typical for all patients or only the sickest.

The next step is to identify the data sources. Most safety projects involve the collection of primary data. There are multiple ways to collect primary data: through self-report, through observations, or through biophysiologic measures. Self-report allows the respondent to document the responses to questions through mechanisms such as surveys, computer-assisted designs, interviews, telephone, or mail. For example, a survey of staff to measure the safety culture of the unit may be administered through interoffice mail via sealed envelopes that can be returned confidentially. An alternative may be an observational study in which a team member observes the work processes and documents his or her findings. For example, if the focus is on infection control, a team member may observe surgical procedures for breaks in aseptic technique. For problems that focus on outcomes of clinical processes, biophysiologic measures such as oxygen saturation, blood pressure, or pulse may provide useful information to measure the patient's response to care (e.g., pain management of moderate sedation). Table 5.4 provides an outline of the specific steps in a patient safety measure plan that can be used to guide the process.

Evaluating Validity and Reliability

The evaluation phase includes estimating the strength of the patient safety measure in the clinical setting, and developing a plan for the analysis. Established patient safety measures will have reported estimates of reliability and validity. If team members are familiar with techniques to assess reliability and validity, then the patient safety measure's estimates can be reviewed by the team. Otherwise, it would be advisable to consult with an expert in measurement or a researcher to assist with the measure selection.

Table 5.4 Patient Safety Measure Plan

Measure Plan	Selected Measure
Patient Safety Measure Selected	Name: Source:
Concepts Included	
Unit of Analysis	❏ Patient ❏ Unit ❏ Organization
Target Sample	Target sample _____ Number of observations _____ Timing of data collection _____ Setting of data collection_____

Data Collection Source	❏ Primary
	    ❏ Self-report
	    ❏ Observation
	    ❏ Biophysiologic
	    ❏ Other_____
	
	❏ Secondary
	    ❏ Chart review
	    ❏ Database
	    ❏ Other_____

Method of Collection	❏ Computer assisted ❏ Mail ❏ Interviews ❏ Written instrument ❏ Telephone
Is Risk Adjustment Required?	❏ Yes (if yes, document methods_____ ❏ No

Responsibility
 	
   Data Collection
 	
   Data Analysis and Reporting
	
	_____
	
	_____

Clinical Staff Involved	❏ RN ❏ MD ❏ UAP ❏ Clerical ❏ Respiratory therapist ❏ Physical therapist ❏ Laboratory
Communication Plan	Date: _____ Audience: _____ Mechanism: ❏ Oral presentation ❏ Video ❏ Written abstract ❏ In-service ❏ Education binder ❏ Committee meeting
Administration Instructions Include	❏ Overview of PI initiative and measure ❏ Clear instructions on how to complete each item ❏ Who to contact if there are questions ❏ Examples, if indicated ❏ Dates and times to be completed ❏ Where to return completed product
Where will the results be reported and when?	Report to:_____ Date:_____

Validity in this context will also involve validating that the clinicians on the team in the patient care area believe that the patient safety measures are important and quantifying the phenomena of interest. The team will need to review the measure to assure that it is consistent with the concept of interest and purpose of the safety project. Table 5.5 can be used to screen patient safety measures.

Table 5.5   Instrument Evaluation

Are concepts consistent with conceptual definitions?	❏ Yes	❏ No
Are there any ethical issues to consider?	❏ Yes	❏ No
Is the reliability estimated and acceptable?	❏ Yes	❏ No
Is the validity estimated and acceptable?	❏ Yes	❏ No
Is the sensitivity estimated and acceptable?	❏ Yes	❏ No
Is the specificity estimated and acceptable?	❏ Yes	❏ No
Is the measure feasible to administer?	❏ Yes	❏ No
Is the measure easy to administer?	❏ Yes	❏ No

Other considerations include review of the sensitivity (positive findings are positive) and specificity (negative findings are negative) of the measure, ease of administration, and if any ethical considerations are associated with the method. The plan for data analysis should also be considered.

This data analysis plan will need to include both the scoring directions and the details of the analysis. The items on an instrument that is in the public domain usually have scoring guidelines to direct their use and interpretation. If scoring guidelines are not available, then the team will need to create a scoring convention.

If the data represent categories (i.e., types of catheters, presence or absence of an item, staff job title), the categories can be defined as names or numbers; for example, if two categories are present and the item measures the presence or absence of a process, then zero is used if the process is not present, and one if it is. If there are three categories, such as reviewing infection rates with the use of three skin prep solutions, each category would be defined by its name, or a designated number (e.g., povidone-iodine paint only = 1, povidone-iodine paint and 5-minute scrub = 2, and iodophor/alcohol single-application film = 3). If the data are continuous, then the scores will usually range from zero or one to the highest score possible in the response format.

Pilot Testing the Measures

The patient safety measure should be piloted to test the clarity, precision, reliability, consistency, meaning adequacy, feasibility, utility, validity, and consensus that the measure is appropriate for the purpose intended (Waltz et al., 1991). This pilot will be conducted using the selected measure with a small number of elements, observations, or responses.

Access to a computer program and the skills to analyze the data—or a resource to provide this service—will be essential to the project planning, as well as the team's ability to interpret and present the results. Hand calculating results is prone to error, and does not give the team the flexibility of looking at results in multiple ways with accompanying graphics. Safety outcomes reports are commonly descriptive in nature, reporting frequencies and means. These statistics are usually supported well with a graphic display of the trends, such as histograms, line graphs or pie charts. Reporting the significance of the change would add a level of rigor, but requires competency in using a statistical program or access to a statistical consultant.

Locating Examples of Measures

There are a variety of internal and external sources of safety measures. Chapter 11 contains a variety of resources that will be helpful in identifying a safety project, planning an intervention, and measuring progress. Within your organization, consider the Performance Improvement or Risk Management department. They will be able to provide you with organizational priorities for safety, so that you can link your initiative to a strategically important effort. Another internal resource is your PI representative or multidisciplinary PI team, who will have access to the safety projects that are being conducted. This will allow you to network with other units who have the same interests. Organizational performance improvement efforts are discussed in more depth in Chapter 2.

Externally, another helpful source is the professional network. Discussions with the professional organization representatives or peers at a professional meeting provide a rich source of ideas and lessons learned. You may also consider doing a search on the HAPI (Health and Psychosocial Instruments) database. Enter the concepts that you would like to study, and HAPI provides a list of instruments for you to review. Another source to consider is a nurse researcher, who may be able to link you to current projects or measures used in completed projects.

Now that the process of selecting measures has been described, the rest of the chapter will focus on a discussion of specific structures, processes, or outcomes that may be of interest to your safety team. These concepts will be further described as they apply to measuring patient safety.

Safety Measures of Structure, Process, and Outcome

To illustrate concepts that can be used in measuring patient safety, the metrics of structure, process, and outcome associated with patient injury will be further discussed. These measures are associated with variations in practice or outcomes, and have been linked to favorable or adverse health of patients, or outcomes.

Should You Measure Structure, Process, or Outcome?

The measure should be selected to match the identified problem and proposed intervention. The choice will depend on the project problem and goal. Is the focus of the problem structure (having the right things), process (doing the right things), or outcomes (having the right things happen)—or a mixture? Table 5.6 describes some common structure, process, and outcome measures.

Table 5.6   Examples of Structure, Process, and Outcome Measures

Structure	Process	Outcome
Compliance with guidelines	Teamwork	Postoperative infection
Mock emergency drills	Continuity of care	Incidence of delirium
Use of screening tools	Medication administration	Complications of surgery
Competency training	Insertion of catheter	Glucose goals
Equipment availability	Transfer of care	Fluid overload
Screening for falls	Aseptic technique	Falls
Number of nurses	Site verification	Return to ICU
Hours per patient day	Blood administration	Incidence of pneumonia

In the vignette at the beginning of the chapter in which the safety strap was missing from the operating room table, the focus may be a structure measure, as in Table 5.7. These structure measures can be linked to processes or outcomes. Nursing structure variables include generic measures such as number of nurses, or nursing hours per patient day (HPPD).

Table 5.7   A Structure Measure for Presence of Equipment in the Operating Room

1. Is safety strap present?	❏ Yes ❏ No

A process measure will use the steps in a standard care protocol to create a template for the best practice. Advantages of process measures include that they measure what we do, can be accomplished within a short time frame, can use small samples, are often unobtrusive, and can be influenced and interpreted by clinicians (McGlynn, 1998). More attention must focus on these processes because safe care is dependent on effective teams, and there is a paucity of methods to monitor team performance (Committee on the Work Environment of Nurses and Patient Safety, 2004). An example of measurement of these processes has evolved as a result of recent errors in wrong-site, wrong-patient, wrong-procedure surgery. The Association of periOperative Registered Nurses (AORN) has developed a Correct Site Surgery ToolKit (available at www.aorn.org/toolkit/nmdefault.asp

Accessed 6/14/04.) These errors have again prompted site verification as a priority in JCAHO goals for 2004 (Joint Commission on Accreditation of Healthcare Organizations, 2003). Process measures would capture the steps in marking the procedure site, so that the specific items that lead to process failure can be further explored, and focused attention can be dedicated to correction of the problem. Table 5.8 demonstrates a potential process measure.

Table 5.8   A Process Measure for Surgical Site Verification in the Operating Room

1. Surgical site is marked.	❑ Yes	❑ No
2. Surgical site marked matches the consent.	❑ Yes	❑ No
3. Patient verified surgical site.	❑ Yes	❑ No
4. Nurse, anesthesiologist, and surgeon paused prior to incision and agreed on surgical site.	❑ Yes	❑ No

Outcome measures reflect the patient response to care, such as achievement of a return to health goal, recovery, improvements in functional status, or survival (Donabedian, 1966). In addition, outcome measures must be important, occur commonly, affect patient care, and be risk adjusted (Iezzoni, 1994). The advantage of using outcomes include that they are significant to patients, represent the goals of clinical care, and can be used across many patient populations (McGlynn, 1998). Important or significant outcomes can emerge from a variety of sources, such as through performance improvement, sentinel events, internal organizational communication or committees, or external sources such as professional, regulatory, or public sources.

Outcomes should occur commonly enough so that data collection will provide the information needed to direct clinical changes. For example, if the outcome of interest was the incidence of catheter-related nosocomial urinary tract infection, and the rate of urinary tract infection was 5%, it would be difficult to monitor changes at the patient or unit level because the outcome is so infrequent. The unit may discharge 600 patients, but only 100 have urethral catheters inserted; of these 100, expecting only 5 infections would make the monitoring of improvements in outcomes difficult.

Risk adjustment, discussed earlier in this chapter, would utilize co-morbidities and/or a severity measure to assure that the variations among patients were controlled for in the analysis. Risk adjustment may be different for each project. These adjustments could be as simple as hours in the operating room for post-operative infection, an acuity measure used on the unit, or co-morbidity ratings. Another approach would be to stratify the patient population into mutually exclusive categories. An example is to use New York Heart Association categories if you were interested in phenomena related to heart failure. Risk adjustment or stratification helps to make the results interpretable, and controls for patient-level differences.

The Agency for Healthcare Research and Quality has provided a set of quality measures for organizational use that have estimates of reliability and validity (Agency for Healthcare Research and Quality, 2003a; Agency for Healthcare Research and Quality, 2003b). In addition, there are also quality initiatives that can be reviewed with specific measures that relate more to care processes. One such effort is The Quality Indicator Project by The Association of Maryland Hospitals & Health Systems (2003), which includes clinical performance measures for acute care, psychiatric care, long-term care, and home care.

It would be remiss to exclude a brief discussion of the recent work on nurse-sensitive outcomes. Nurse-sensitive outcomes (patient responses that have significant relationships to nursing care) have included mortality, medication errors, failure to rescue, urinary tract infection, and patient complications (see Table 5.9). To the extent possible, nurses should include nurse-sensitive measures in safety projects, so that their effect on patient outcomes can be evaluated, improved, and communicated. Through their Safety and Quality Initiative, the American Nurses Association has developed a number of nationally used nurse-sensitive indicators in the National Database of Nursing Quality Indicators (NDNQI) (ANA's Safety & Quality Initiative, 2003) that are available for review.

Table 5.9 Nurse-Sensitive Outcomes

Aiken et al. (1994; 2002; 2003)	Mortality
Blegen et al. (1998)	Medication errors, decubiti, and patient complaints
Dang, Pronovost et al. (2002)	Surgical complications
Kovner et al. (1998; 2002)	Urinary tract infection, pulmonary compromise, and thrombosis
Needleman et al. (2001; 2002)	Failure to rescue, urinary tract infection, and pneumonia.
Unruh (2003)	Decubiti, pneumonia

Nurses have diverse opportunities to focus on structures, processes, and outcomes to improve patient safety. The focus of study will depend on the problem identified within the team or clinical unit. Multiple examples and resources have been discussed to begin to highlight patient safety measures that can be used in safety projects. Patient safety measures are associated with variations in clinical practice or outcomes, and have been linked to adverse patient outcomes.

Conclusion

Becoming involved in safety projects requires that nurses partner with other multidisciplinary team members to approach problems as a system of care. Choosing the right measure in a safety project allows the team to interpret the impact of the intervention. Nurses are in a unique position to be involved in safety projects because they are intimately familiar with what systems have and don't have (structures), and what systems do and don't do (processes). Measurement of safety outcomes will require that nurses become familiar with measuring what we get as a product from our care for patients based on the resources that we have and the actions that we take.

Measuring patient safety is an essential skill for nurse leaders. It is how they communicate internally to colleagues such as physicians, pharmacists, and respiratory therapists. Measurement is also a method of communication externally to accrediting agencies, legislators, and other professionals regarding the value nurses add to patient care. Strong competency in measuring patient safety will enhance the nurse's value as an essential member of the healthcare improvement team.

References

Agency for Healthcare Research and Quality. (2003a). AHRQ quality indicators. Retrieved June 13, 2004, from http://www.qualityindicators.ahrq.gov/data/hcup/qinext.htm

Agency for Healthcare Research and Quality. (2003b). Patient safety indicators. Retrieved June 13, 2004. from http://www.qualityindicators.ahrq.gov/data/hcup/psi.htm

Aiken, L. H. (1994). Good nursing care = lower death rates. *N. J. Nurse, 24,* 1.

Aiken, L. H., Smith, H. L., & Lake, E. T. (1994). Lower Medicare mortality among a set of hospitals known for good nursing care. *Medical Care, 32,* 771–787.

Aiken, L. H., Clarke, S. P., Sloane, D. M., Sochalski, J., & Silber, J. H. (2002). Hospital nurse staffing and patient mortality, nurse burnout, and job dissatisfaction. *Journal of the American Medical Association, 288,* 1987–1993.

Aiken, L. H., Clarke, S. P., Cheung, R. B., Sloane, D. M., & Silber, J. H. (2003). Educational levels of hospital nurses and surgical patient mortality. *Journal of the American Medical Association, 290,* 1617–1623.

American Nurses Association's (ANA) Safety & Quality Initiative. (2003). National database of nursing quality indicators (NDNQI). Retrieved June 13, 2004, from http://www.mriresearch.org/researchservices/healthsciences/ndnqi/ndnqi.asp

American Society of Anesthesiologists. (2003). ASA physical status classification system. Retrieved June 13, 2004, from http://www.asahq.org/clinical/physicalstatus.htm

Association of Maryland Hospitals & Health Systems. (2003). Learn about the QI Project. Retrieved from http://www.qiproject.org

Berens, M. J. (2002, July 23). Drug-resistant germs adapt, thrive beyond hospital walls. *Chicago Tribune,* page 1.

Berwick, D. M. (1996). A primer on leading the improvement of systems. *British Journal of Medicine, 312,* 619–622 (9 March).

Berwick, D. M., James, B., & Coye, M. J. (2003). Connections between quality measurement and improvement. *Medical Care, 41,* I-30–I-38.

Blegan, M. A., Goode, C. J., & Reed, L. (1998). Nurse staffing and patient outcomes. *Nursing Research, 47* (1), 43–50.

Committee on Quality of Health Care in America, Institute of Medicine. (1999). To err is human: Building a safer health system. Retrieved from http://books.nap.edu/html/to_err_is_human/exec_summ.html

Committee on Quality of Health Care in America, I.O.M. (2001). *Crossing the quality chasm: A new health system for the 21st century.* Washington, DC: The National Academies Press.

Committee on the Work Environment of Nurses and Patient Safety. (2004). *Keeping patients safe: Transforming the work environment of nurses.* Washington, DC: The National Academies Press.

Dang, D., Johantgen, M. E., Pronovost, P. J., Jenckes, M. W., & Bass, E. B. (2002). Postoperative complications: does intensive care unit staff nursing make a difference? *Heart Lung, 31,* 219–228.

Donabedian, A. (1966). Evaluating the quality of medical care. *Milbank Memorial Fund Quarterly, 44* (part 2), 166–206.

Donabedian, A. (1985). *The methods and findings of quality assessment and monitoring: An illustrated analysis,* Health Administration Press Series: Explorations in quality assessment and monitoring (vol. 3). Ann Arbor, MI.

Iezzoni, L. I. (1994). Using risk-adjusted outcomes to assess clinical practice: An overview of issues pertaining to risk adjustment. *Annals of Thoracic Surgery, 58,* 1822–1826.

Joint Commission on Accreditation of Healthcare Organizations. (2003). 2004 national patient safety goals. Retrieved from http://www.jcaho.org/accredited+organizations/patient+safety/04+npsg/04_npsg.htm

Kinzer, K. W. (2001). Patient safety: A call to action: A consensus statement from the National Quality Forum. *Medscape General Medicine, 3.* Available at: http://www.medscape.com/Medscape/General Medicine/journal/2001/v03.n02/mgm0321.01.kinze/mgm03

Kovner, C. & Gergen, P. J. (1998). Nurse staffing levels and adverse effects following surgery in U.S. hospitals. *Image: Journal of Nursing Scholarship, 30,* 315–321.

Kovner, C., Jones, C., Zhan, C., Gergen, P. J., & Basu, J. (2002). Nurse staffing and postsurgical adverse events: an analysis of administrative data from a sample of U.S. hospitals, 1990-1996. *Health Services Research, 37,* 611–629.

McGlynn, E. A. (1998). Choosing and evaluating clinical performance measures. *The Joint Commission Journal on Quality Improvement, 24,* 470–479.

McGlynn, E. A. (2003). Selecting common measures of quality and system performance. *Medical Care, 41,* 139–147.

Merriam-Webster's Collegiate Dictionary (10th ed.). (1996). Springfield, MA: Merriam-Webster.

Miller, M. R., Elixhauser, A., & Zhan, C. (2003). Patient safety events during pediatric hospitalizations. *Pediatrics, 111,* 1358–1366.

Miller, M. R., Elixhauser, A., Zhan, C., & Meyer, G. S. (2001). Patient safety indicators: Using administrative data to identify potential patient safety concerns. *Health Services Research, 36,* 110–132.

Moen, R. D. & Pronovost, P. J. (2003). *Quality measurement: A practical guide for the ICU.* Marblehead, MA: HCPro.

Needleman, J., Buerhaus, P. I., Mattke, S., Stewart, M., & Zelevinsky, K. (2001). Nurse staffing and patient outcomes in hospitals (*Rep. No. US Department of Health and Human Services, Health Resources and Services Administration 230-99-0021*). Boston, MA: Harvard School of Public Health.

Needleman, J., Buerhaus, P., Mattke, S., Stewart, M., & Zelevinsky, K. (2002). Nurse-staffing levels and the quality of care in hospitals. *New England Journal of Medicine, 346,* 1715–1722.

Polit, D. F., Beck, C. T., & Hungler, B. P. (2001). *Essentials of nursing research methods, appraisal, and utilization* (5th ed.). Philadelphia: Lippincott.

Polit, D. F. & Beck, C. T. (2004). *Nursing Research Principles and Methods.* (7th ed.) Baltimore: Lippincott Williams & Wilkins.

Pronovost, P. J., Miller, M. R., Dorman, T., Berenholtz, S., Rubin, H. (2001). Developing and implementing measures of quality of care in the intensive care unit. *Current Opinion in Critical Care, 7,* 297–303.

Pronovost, P. J. & Berenholtz, S. M. (2002). *Practical guide to measuring performance in the intensive care unit.* Irving, TX: VHA.

Pronovost, P. J. & Berenholtz, S. M. (2004). *Improving sepsis care in the intensive care unit: An evidence-based approach.* Irving, TX: VHA.

Solberg, L. I., Mosser, G., & McDonald, S. (1997). The three faces of performance measurement: Improvement, accountability, and research. *Journal on Quality Improvement, 23,* 135–147.

Unruh, L. (2003). Licensed nurse staffing and adverse events in hospitals. *Medical Care, 41,* 142–152.

Waltz, C. F., Strickland, O. L., & Lenz, E. R. (1991). *Measurement in nursing research.* Philadelphia: F.A. Davis.

CHAPTER 6

Dissemination of Findings

Dina A. Krenzischek, MAS, RN, CPAN*

Robin P. Newhouse, Ph.D., RN†

A post-anesthesia care unit (PACU) nurse pricked her finger with a capillary tube after completing hematocrit testing on a patient with hepatitis. She was seriously concerned that she was at risk to acquire hepatitis. Fortunately, she did not. This incident did, however, heighten awareness of a problem. Because of the importance of providing the safest equipment for nurses to use, a market search was done to replace the current system. Offering point-of-care testing for patients preoperatively is an efficient and effective way to screen patients for surgery. Laboratory experts and post-anesthesia nurses collaborated to review options for a safer device. The laboratory tested the selected device and approved its utilization in the PACU area. After staff training and protocol implementation with the new equipment, nurses became suspicious of the accuracy of hemoglobin values. The results seemed unusually low or inconsistent with the clinical assessment. A review of the problem found that individual variations in the protocol affect accurate hemoglobin results. These variations could lead to inaccurate assessment of patients in the PACU.

In this situation, the nurse leaders identified the need to collaborate with the lab to select a product that was feasible and safe for nurses to use and that produced accurate lab values to provide safe patient care. Meeting this goal required internal communication and subsequent dissemination of lessons learned to other clinicians who may be using the same device. Dissemination

*Nurse Manager
 The Johns Hopkins Hospital

†Nurse Researcher/Assistant Professor
 The Johns Hopkins Hospital/The Johns Hopkins University School of Nursing

of performance improvement and research findings, research utilization, and evidence-based practices have become increasingly more important (Gillis, 2002). Important results that apply to other settings or organizations should be disseminated not only within the organization, but also to the public sector. Nurses have a role in this dissemination of knowledge.

Nurses provide testimonies, participate in governmental hearings, and serve on committees, task forces, and commissions related to health care. They participate in teleconferences, development of web sites, videos, and radio and television shows. Nurses in all settings are involved in the development of technological innovations such as computerized documentation systems, electronic databases, and institutional web sites, and have become proficient in the use of e-mail and the Internet. These efforts have demanded skill expansion as nurses work in teams and disseminate information.

To disseminate findings of safety projects and research, it is important to: 1) identify the appropriate audience who can apply or change practice, and 2) use resources that can support the implementation of such a change. To explore these areas, the objectives of this chapter are to:

- Describe the internal and external organizational dissemination processes
- Identify opportunities for presentation of safety project outcomes
- Discuss successful presentation strategies.

Internal and External Dissemination

Findings can be disseminated internally within the institution or facility, and externally outside the institution. Internally, dissemination is necessary to influence changes in practice, policy, procedure, and protocol as a result of safety project findings. It is important to share lessons learned not only within the unit or work area, but also with other units that may have a similar patient population. Institutionally, it is imperative to review the implications of the results of projects so that as best practices are implemented, the standard of care is similar within the organization. External dissemination is also an important force to broaden the influence of best practices.

Methods of dissemination of findings can vary, but are similar for both internal and external dissemination. Internally, presentation to the target group is the most common method of dissemination. Information can be communicated by memo, flyers, educational materials, abstracts, posters, or oral presentation. The use of e-mail, web sites, and the Internet is growing as nurses increasingly use technology to communicate.

These same mechanisms can be used externally through the professional network nationally and internationally.

Internal Dissemination

Internal dissemination results in communication of lessons learned within the organization. Internal organizational communication begins with a communication plan. The patient safety project leader should first discuss the project with, and seek advice from, the Director of Nursing (DON), Vice President of Patient Care Services (VP), or the designee for safety projects. Internal dissemination efforts need to be coordinated by leadership for effective communication that includes all stakeholders. The DON or VP can link the safety project to the organizational safety plan, assuring strategic importance. These people are ultimately responsible for organizational patient safety within their scope of responsibility, which includes the implementation of new practices and approval of policy, procedure, and protocols. The meeting with the DON or VP should include discussions of the following topics related to dissemination: the target audience, goals, timing, methods, cost, and communication pathway and plan. The implications to other departments should be considered. Plans for external dissemination should also be included, if appropriate.

In the hemoglobin example at the beginning of the chapter, the project grew from a unit-based to a departmental implementation. Committees involved in practice standards, performance improvement, and education needed to become involved. A collaborative effort ensued between the departments of surgery and anesthesiology, and the hematology laboratory. This collaboration resulted in a more structured point-of-care testing program that was redesigned to meet all the needs of the functional clinical departments as well as the laboratory regulatory requirements. Dissemination of findings to other departments enhanced cooperation and resulted in efficient implementation of corrective strategies.

Not all safety project outcomes have limited application to the internal or organizational level. Some projects should have wider dissemination because of the scope of the impact or the wider application. These projects should be disseminated externally.

External Dissemination

There are multiple external opportunities for nurses to disseminate the results of safety projects. At the local level, specialty organizations have monthly meetings and various educational offerings. At the national level, poster and oral presentations are advertised annually for national and international conferences. There are also opportunities to work on professional guidelines, task forces, committees, or publication of manuscripts in journals. Dissemination through abstracts, oral presentations, poster presentation, and publication are all mechanisms of external dissemination. An abstract is often the first step in submitting a proposal for a poster or oral presentation.

Submitting the Abstract

An abstract is a synopsis of the research plan or project that briefly summarizes the study objectives, methods, and expected results (Mateo & Kirchhoff, 1999). It is common for conference organizers to call for abstracts for poster, oral, panel, or symposium presentations. Before developing the abstract, the author should obtain the abstract template or requirements from the organization's newsletter, web site, or main office. These requirements will include the abstract headings, the total number of words allowed, and deadlines. Usual elements include the problem, research questions, hypotheses, conceptual framework, methods, results, conclusions, and implications. The abstract usually is peer reviewed for recommendations for acceptance. Peer review means that experts in the field review the content for appropriateness for the intended presentation. It is customary to receive notification that the abstract submission has been received. Follow-up with the sponsoring organization may be necessary if verification of receipt of the submission is not received prior to the submission deadline.

Before submitting for an oral or poster presentation, authors must take into account many considerations (Mateo & Kirchhoff, 1999) (see Table 6.1). First, consider the conference objectives, and how your project fits with these objectives. You will need to review the categories in the call for abstracts and presentations. Next, determine the conference date, time, and location, and make sure they match your availability. Knowledge of the location will help you plan for the costs of travel and lodging. Travel, meals, registration, and accommodations are major expenses in attending a conference. Travel by air, train, bus, or car are options with a wide range of costs and time required to reach the destination. Accommodation cost can be decreased by sharing a room with colleagues or contacting the main office of the organization to inquire if they have a list of members looking for a roommate. An additional cost is conference registration, which is often a requirement for presenters.

Table 6.1 Considerations Before Submitting an Abstract

Conference date, time, and location
Cost of travel, accommodation, registration, and meals
Source of funding
Target audience
Conference objectives

Next consider the source of funding. Determine if your institution supports employees who are conducting professional presentations. If they do not cover the total expense, determine which portion of the cost, if any, can be reimbursed to you. Some organizations have scholarship programs available to members to supplement presentation costs. Also consider professional organization sponsorship. Make sure to explore the options well ahead of time, and understand the process and the required document submission.

The last point is to understand the target audience. The content of the presentation should be individualized to the conference topic and audience. Some conferences organize their topics into levels from basic to advanced, so the content needs to be adjusted to the indicated level. It is helpful to use the objectives of the conference to guide the development of your presentation.

Beyond submitting the abstract, there are a number of additional considerations depending on whether you intend to present an oral or a poster presentation. Oral presentations will be covered next.

Oral Presentations

Oral presentations require special considerations, including time, method of delivery, technology support, and logistics. When creating the plan for your oral presentation, first determine the total amount of time allotted. Basic considerations for oral presentations can be reviewed in Table 6.2.

Table 6.2 Considerations for Oral Presentations

Category	Description
Time	Verify the time frame of the presentation. Practice and adjust content to fit within the allowed time. Allow time for a question and answer period within the time frame.
Method	Determine format (PowerPoint, color, type of graphics). Distribute handouts. A copy of the PowerPoint presentation with note taking space is preferred. Make copies of the abstract for attendees, if required.
Technology	Consider slide tray and request slide projector. Consider computer with PowerPoint presentation. Check PowerPoint cables and extension cord. Check type of drive (e.g., floppy disk, CD, Zip). Determine whether AV support is available. Choose microphone: stationary or attached to the outfit of the presenter. Go to speaker ready room to check presentation.
Logistics	Check the height of the podium. Request an additional table for the computer, if needed. Keep notes on questions because it can enhance future presentations. Provide business card upon request. Determine the travel time to the conference room. Determine the size of the room. Determine the potential number of people in the audience. Visit the conference room before the presentation.

Time.   Usually, several speakers present within a specific time frame. Create an outline of your presentation based on your objectives that fits within the allowed time. Determine who will be presenting if there is more than one author. A conversation with the team up front prevents team conflict later. If your presentation abstract is accepted for oral presentation, your planning is not done. You will need to complete the conference speaker information, and return your letter of acceptance 3 to 6 months before the conference date. The speaker notification packet will come with or be followed by specific information for presenters. This information needs to be completed within the designated time, and will include requests for items such as a content outline, conflict of interest statement, honorarium agreements, travel arrangements, or a biosketch.

Method.   The second issue is the method of delivery. Refine the outline and create audiovisual supports for your presentation. You will need to practice the presentation to time the content, adjusting it to fit within the allowed time frame. Fifteen minutes is usually allocated for content presentation and five minutes for questions. Choose the format for audiovisuals, color scheme, and type of graphics needed, and determine if handouts are expected. The sponsoring organization may publish handouts in the conference proceedings, and request that no handouts be provided. Also, determine if the abstract will be available in the conference proceedings, or if you need to provide it for participants. For the audiovisuals, some conference organizers provide a PowerPoint template with a color scheme. Others allow the presenter to create their own. Adhere to the specific rules established by the sponsor.

Technology.   Another issue is to determine the type of technology required and available. The information packet will include the types of audiovisual equipment available (e.g., slide projector, overhead projector, PowerPoint) and computer needs. Ask if a computer is available or if you will need to provide your own. If one is available, determine the type of drive so that you can prepare your presentation in the correct format (e.g., floppy disk, CD, Zip).

You will also need to determine the type of audio equipment that will be provided to you as a speaker, such as a microphone or podium. A microphone can be stationary or attached to the clothing of the presenter.

Logistics.   Logistics include the room size and location, time needed to travel between locations, and some considerations related to the presentation itself. You will need to determine the location and size of the room, as well as the travel time required to get to the presentation conference room from your previous destination. The size of the room will give you an idea of the number of participants that conference planners expect to attend your session. Visit the room before the presentation so that you feel more comfortable with the setup, and can adjust the presentation plan if needed.

Check the room, and observe the height of the podium. Depending on your height, you may need to request a podium or microphone adjustment.

An additional table can be requested for a computer if needed. Determine where you will place your handouts, if used.

During the presentation, plan to make note of the questions raised, so that you can enhance future presentations. Also remember to bring business cards or contact information for interested attendees.

An oral presentation often helps presenters to organize thoughts around specific objectives. This refinement can then act as a template from which to construct a manuscript for publication. The feedback from the audience is valuable in considering ways to improve the project, how others experience the same problem, and how to further expand or review the practice, theory, or research implications of your work. Poster presentations can also serve as a mechanism to disseminate your safety project, while providing an interactive networking session with other conference attendees.

Poster Presentation

A poster presentation requires similar preparation as the steps discussed for oral presentations (see Table 6.3). An abstract is submitted and reviewed, and the author is notified of rejection or acceptance. Just as in an oral presentation, the presenter will need to check the location and time for presentation. The difference for the poster presentation is in the method of presentation and the details of constructing the poster.

Table 6.3   Considerations for Poster Presentations

Category	Description
Time	Verify poster setup, presentation, and take-down time. Keep notes on questions or suggestions to enhance future work or presentations.
Location	Determine the presentation room and poster location.

Type of display	Select bulletin board or table and size:
	    Table: use stand-alone tabletop display.
	    Bulletin board: usually 4 × 8 feet.
	Establish poster and plan layout.
	Select type of media and size.

Layout	Decide on the layout of information to be presented. Adhere to the sponsoring agency or organization's guidelines for posters.
Other considerations	Decide how the paper will be mounted and bring necessary materials such as pins or Velcro.

The first consideration is the type of display. Determine if the display format is a bulletin board or table top, and the size specifications. If a table is provided, you will use a stand-alone tabletop display. If a bulletin board will be used, the size is usually 4 feet by 8 feet. This will help plan the layout of the poster.

Next, choose the size and media. Poster sizes of 4 feet by 8 feet will usually take up all of the bulletin board space provided. A smaller poster of 3 feet by 6 feet may be adequate to present your safety project. The media used may be paper or plastic. Numerous vendors have services available to create posters for a fee. Presenters can prepare the poster in a PowerPoint document, using instructions for the font and layout provided by the vendor. Be sure to ask the vendor when they need your document; when the draft will be ready; and once approved, when the poster will be ready and the price.

The next step is to prepare the poster. Determine the poster layout and the information to be presented. Some practical tips include:

- Adhere to the guidelines established by the sponsoring organization.
- Keep it simple, concise, and organized.
- Use a font and format that are readable from 3–5 feet.
- Use color, graphs, and pictures.
- Highlight significant points by using bullets and asterisks.
- Design the poster to be easily understood within 5 minutes.
- Guide readers by using directional lines, and headings and subheadings in bold print.
- Bring the necessary materials to hang the poster (e.g., pins, Velcro).

Allow ample time to view the draft poster before the final printing, based on your vendor's instructions. This will allow changes if needed, and avoid an unnecessary expense of reprinting the poster. Pick the poster up, and plan to carry it in a protective case that can be easily transported.

At the conference, place your poster at the designated place at the time and date requested by the conference sponsors. It is usually the day before the conference opens to one-half to one hour before the poster session opening. Keep your poster up for the length of time indicated for the poster session, and plan to stand by your poster so that attendees can view your project and ask questions. Remember to take your business cards and any handouts that you want to provide to attendees. Take down the poster at the required time.

Poster presentations provide an opportunity to highlight completed or ongoing projects, network with a high volume of interested colleagues, engage in a dialogue with others who are conducting similar work, and exchange contact information. There are some advantages to presenting a poster instead of giving an oral presentation, including not needing a detailed presentation outline, not preparing audiovisuals, not having to time the presentation to fit in an allotted period, and not having to practice the oral presentation. Beyond presenting posters or oral sessions, publication is another way to widely disseminate lessons learned.

Publication

Publishing safety projects through print or electronic media provides one of the most visible and accessible means to widely disseminate lessons learned in safety projects. Publications are archived and retrievable through multiple literature review search engines. Publications then reach not only the subscribers of the journal, but also wider audiences searching for specific topics. Taking the extra step to publish a manuscript for a safety project can impact patient safety internationally and link safety teams tackling similar problems.

De Back (2001), editor of *International Nursing Review,* discussed the basic steps in publishing a manuscript. These steps were:

1. Plan the article.
2. Gather the data.
3. Develop an objective statement.
4. Describe the scope of the article.
5. Describe the significance of the project of study.
6. Develop supporting tables and figures.
7. Write conclusions and implications.
8. Summarize references.

As you plan the article, target a specific journal for submission of your publication. A letter of intent or query will help to determine the journal's interest in the topic, and may provide guidance on the article's purpose or content. The editor may want a specific presentation style or recommend a redirection of the focus of the manuscript. This information will facilitate the process and avoid some frustrations as a result of unclear expectations.

Check the journal or web site for guidelines for publication. These guidelines will be helpful for framing your article. A checklist may also be available for authors to follow. Take some time to review the content of the journal, so that you can be comfortable with the style of writing and the reader's interest. Review similar articles to get a sense of the flow of the text. You will need to become familiar with the editorial style and reference format. Developing an objective statement for the manuscript will help to keep you focused on what content should be included. Then describe the scope of the article and the significance of the project. Outline the body of your article with the supporting literature, including your conclusions and implications for practice.

Title, author names, and affiliation.   These are usually presented first. The title should speak clearly to what the article is about including design, participants or phenomena, and variables. The primary author's name appears first and then the secondary authors. The primary author or team will need to discuss how subsequent authors will be listed. Potential options include alphabetical listing or listing authors in descending order according to the amount of effort contributed by each co-author.

Problem and brief background. The problem must be clearly stated. Describe what is known and who are affected, what factors contribute to the existing problem, and when these problems occur. A literature review is used to further extend the state of the knowledge on the topic, and identify gaps in the literature. The conceptual framework presents the context for studying the problem and can be viewed as a map for understanding relationships between or among the variables (Miller, 2002).

Purpose and goal of the article. The purpose of the study should include the aim of the research, target population, setting, and research variables (Mateo & Kirchhoff, 1999). If the safety project is research based, research questions or hypotheses should be included.

Methodology. The methodology is a description of how the project was conducted. It describes the design, participants, how the subjects were selected, where the study will occur, how the data was collected, what type of evaluation tools were used, and how the data was analyzed.

Results. The results section presents your data in narrative and table format. Start with descriptive data, then move to inferential statistics, if used.

Discussion and implications. Discuss the lessons learned through your project, and the clinical changes planned or made as a result. Extend the discussion to additional implications for practice, education, or research.

Abstract. A brief abstract (usually no more than 300 words), which summarizes the project, is usually required. The journal format for abstracts should be used.

The manuscript will need to be typed and double spaced. Follow the journal's guidelines on citations and references formats, text, tables, and illustrations. The rule of thumb is that a reference should be less than 5 years old, unless it is a classic article.

After you have completed your draft, give it to a friend to read and critique. Make the revisions and read the manuscript again. When the manuscript is ready to submit, use the checklist provided by the journal to assure that all points are covered before mailing the manuscript. Include a cover letter that introduces the editor to the article and how it relates to her readers' interests. Specify the article title and author(s)' names, home and work address, telephone numbers, and e-mail addresses. Make sure that you have had the manuscript reviewed and approved by the appropriate representative from your institution according to the organizational policy before you submit it to the journal. Send it to the journal address listed in the information for authors or the checklist.

When the manuscript is received by the editor, she will screen it for appropriateness and quality (Sullivan, 2002a). If it is acceptable, it is sent to reviewers, who critique the article and recommend publishing, revising, or not publishing. This process is scheduled to take one month, but is often extended. The reviewers also offer comments to guide revisions. Expect a request for revisions when you get your manuscript back from the editor. You will receive the reviewer comments so that you can revise the content if you agree with the recommendations. Changes are at your discretion; however, acceptance of the article for publication may be affected if you choose not to accept the reviewers' suggestions. After the revisions, read the article again, and then send the final manuscript back to the editor. The article will be re-reviewed, and you will receive notification of acceptance, more revisions, or rejection.

Although journals want to promote publication, manuscripts are sometimes rejected (Sullivan, 2002b). The most frequent reasons relate to:

- Submitted to wrong journal
- No new information provided
- Outdated information
- Narrow topic
- References out of date or missing important contributions
- Reliance on the literature
- Class paper submitted
- Methodology limited or has flaws
- Poor writing

If the manuscript is accepted for publication, the author(s) will be asked to sign a copyright release. Communication from the publisher will occur again after the final edit, and a proof will be sent for approval.

Publication is a powerful vehicle for dissemination of findings for safety project, so prepare, plan, remember to use your peer network to review your work, use the reviewer comments to revise your article, and follow the journal guidelines for publication.

Comparative Study between Bedside and Laboratory Hemoglobin Testing

Both internal and external dissemination of findings were used in the case study at the beginning of this chapter. Internally, both staff nurses and clinical technicians received education on techniques for obtaining blood samples and testing of hemoglobin. Education included the importance of proper technique, and reinforcement that improper technique might result in a low false reading. Research demonstrated that there was a significant positive correlation in hemoglobin results obtained by bedside nurses and laboratory technicians who used the approved guidelines by the Department of Hematology.

From an institutional perspective, the bedside hemoglobin laboratory testing program became the responsibility of nursing in collaboration with the Department of Hematology. The institution continuously improves the systematic PI approach in managing bedside laboratory testing. The new practice was adopted not only in the authors' work location, but also other areas that used the same hemoglobin testing procedure. Some of the major benefits of the centralized implementation of findings were stronger management support from hospital leaders; standardized policies, procedures, and performance improvement activities; and a systematic method of obtaining supplies and equipment, thus reducing the hospital's cost. In addition, the research findings were disseminated using grand rounds presentations and other educational opportunities within the institution.

Externally, an abstract of the project was submitted to the American Society of PeriAnesthesia Nurses (ASPAN) and accepted for poster and oral presentations at the ASPAN National Conference (Krenzischek & Tanseco, 1994). A journal article was subsequently published (Krenzischek & Tanseco, 1996).

Conclusion

In summary, dissemination of findings is no longer a "nice thing to do," but is now a professional obligation for nurse leaders to share findings from safety projects. This chapter discussed the internal and external channels used to disseminate findings, and strategies for successful presentations and publications. A case study was presented that highlighted the importance of the dissemination of findings. The resulting practice improvement was shared through oral and poster presentation at a national convention so that other organizations could learn from the safety project.

Nurses who participate in and lead safety projects can have a broader impact on influencing practice changes by disseminating lessons learned both internally and externally. Building dissemination skills will promote sharing of lessons learned in safety projects, and increase the visibility of the nurse's role in improving safe care for patients.

References

De Back, V. (2001). *Writing for publication.* Presented at the ICN Congress, Copenhagen, Denmark.

Gillis, A. (2002). *Research for nurses: Methods and interpretation.* Philadelphia: F. A. Davis.

Krenzischek, D., & Tanseco, F. (1994). *Comparative study of bedside and laboratory measurements of hemoglobin.* American Society of PeriAnesthesia Nurses. Poster presentation at Atlanta, GA.

Krenzischek, D., & Tanseco, F. (1996). Comparative study of bedside and laboratory measurements of hemoglobin. *American Journal of Critical Care Nurse, 5*(6), 427–432.

LoBlondo-Wood, G., & Hber, J. (2002), Nursing research: Methods, critical appraisal, and utilization. St. Louis: Mosby.

Mateo, M., & Kirchhoff, K. (1999). *Using and conducting nursing research in the clinical setting,* (2nd ed.). Philadelphia: W. B. Saunders.

Miller, B. (2002). *Literature Review in Nursing Research: Methods, Critical Appraisal & Utilization by Wood & Maber;* St. Louis: Mosby, Chapter 4, 77–105.

Sullivan, E. J. (2002a). The manuscript review process. *Journal of Professional Nursing, 18,* 57–58.

Sullivan, E. J. (2002b). Top 10 reasons a manuscript is rejected. *Journal of Professional Nursing, 18,* 1–2.

Tornquist, E. (1999). *From proposal to publication.* Menlo Park, CA: Addison-Wesley.

CHAPTER 7

Safer Care for Patients on Mechanical Ventilation

Sean Berenholtz* MD, MHS
Todd Dorman+# MD
Pedro Mendez-Tellez*, MD

As charge nurse, you routinely do rounds on all patients on your busy medical intensive care unit. The physician member of your team recently mentioned that the incidence of ventilator-associated pneumonia appears to be on the rise. Today on rounds you notice that most of the mechanically ventilated patients on the unit are either in a supine position or have the head of the bed elevated 15 degrees. You have read that the head of the bed should be elevated at least 30 degrees in mechanically ventilated patients. At change of shift report, you mention this fact to a co-worker and discuss ways to change practice without challenging the competence of your team members.

Opportunities to improve care in the intensive care unit (ICU) are considerable. Intensive care is associated with significant morbidity, mortality, and costs, representing an ideal focus for improvement efforts (Angus et al., 2000; Donchin et al., 1995; Halpern, Bettes, & Greenstein, 1994). In addition, it is estimated that on average all of the 5 million patients admitted to adult ICUs suffer a serious preventable adverse event every day (Andrew et al., 1997; Angus et al., 2000). The cost of such events, in both human and financial terms, is high. Intensive care is expensive, accounting for approximately 30% of acute hospital costs, or $180 billion annually (Halpern et al., 1994). Prolonging intensive care due to adverse events, many of which are preventable,

*Assistant Professor, +Associate Professor
Department of Anesthesiology and Critical Care Medicine
The Johns Hopkins University School of Medicine
#The Johns Hopkins School of Nursing

significantly increases the human and financial burden for the unfortunate patient and his or her family. The objective of this chapter is to demonstrate how we applied the principles of quality measurement and improvement to improve the care of mechanically ventilated patients. This "real world" example highlights how we adopted principles from aviation, including strategies to reduce complexity and create redundancy to improve safety. Lessons learned during this endeavor have helped us to improve subsequent care processes.

What Was Our Goal?

Mechanical ventilation is common in the ICU, and is associated with significant morbidity, mortality, and costs of care (Kollef, 1999). There is a rapidly growing body of evidence to guide practice in critical care settings related to the care of mechanically ventilated patients. Several therapies or processes can reduce this burden, including head of bed (HOB) elevation (Drakulovic et al., 1999), peptic ulcer disease (PUD) prophylaxis (Cook et al., 1998), deep venous thrombosis (DVT) prophylaxis (Attia et al., 2001), and holding sedation such that patients can follow commands once a day (Kress et al., 2000). Despite this evidence, a gap exists between available evidence and best practice (Cook et al., 2002). Evidence regarding best practices in the care of mechanically ventilated patients is derived from well-done randomized controlled trials, so the results suggest that if we provide these therapies to our patients, we can expect to see improvements in patient outcomes, including reductions in morbidity, mortality and cost of care.

When examining adherence to these guidelines as part of a collaborative with 11 hospitals, including 13 medical and surgical ICUs, sponsored by the Institute for Healthcare Improvement (IHI) and the VHA, Inc.; in less than 65% of ventilator days did patients receive all four processes (Pronovost et al., 2003). Importantly, performance at some hospitals was >90% for each process, but significant variation in practice existed among hospitals. Based on the median performance from the collaborative and using estimates of efficacy for each of these care processes from the literature, an average ICU with 1,000 admissions per year may be able to prevent 23 deaths and save an additional $2.3 million dollars annually simply by ensuring that patients receive these four evidence-based processes (Pronovost et al., 2003). If we assume an average mortality of 10% for U.S. ICUs (Zimmerman et al., 1998), preventing 23 deaths represents a 23% reduction in mortality for an average ICU with 1,000 admissions per year—a larger impact than for new more expensive therapies to treat sepsis (Bernard et al., 2001). Indeed, these results suggest that one of the most cost effective opportunities to improve patient outcomes in the ICU over the next quarter century may likely come not from discovering new therapies, but from discovering how to deliver therapies that are known to be effective.

How Would We Know When We Reached Our Goal?

In choosing what we should measure, we considered several published criteria (Rubin, Pronovost, & Diette, 2001). First, the area to be improved was determined to be important to the intended audience. By concentrating on the care of mechanically ventilated patients, we were focusing on structural or process measures that might have a significant impact on ICU patient morbidity, mortality, and/or cost of care.

Second, it was important to select measures where the evidence regarding the association between the process or structure and outcome was strong. In considering the strength of the evidence, we considered the type and number of studies available to guide practice. Randomized clinical trials (RCT) provide the strongest level of evidence, whereas observational studies and consensus groups provide significantly weaker evidence. Multiple studies or a meta-analysis of well-done RCTs provide stronger evidence than single studies (Sackett et al., 1996). The strength of the evidence for the measure will determine the likelihood that improvement in the quality measure will produce consistent and credible improvements in quality of care (Brook, McGlynn, & Cleary, 1996; McGlynn, 1998). For example, it is unclear that providing hospitals data on mortality, without data on how to reduce mortality, will lead to improved quality of care. Evidence-based therapies have only recently become available in critical care. For example, we now have evidence that ventilator strategies, tight glucose control, and the use of activated protein C (process measures) are associated with hospital mortality (Berenholtz et al., 2002; Bernard et al., 2001; van den Berghe et al., 2001), and that length of stay can be reduced by daily interruption in sedative-drug infusions (Kress et al., 2000). These may represent appropriate areas for future measures of quality and safety. For the purposes of our mechanical ventilation project, we chose four evidence-based process measures: head of bed elevation, PUD prophylaxis, DVT prophylaxis, and holding sedation.

Third, we evaluated whether variability in performance existed related to performance of these four processes in the care of mechanically ventilated patients in our ICU. Variability represents the potential opportunity for improvement (McGlynn, 1998; McGlynn & Asch, 1998). Indeed, providers may not want to focus on improving rates of catheter-related blood stream infections (CR-BSI) if the rate is already low (below 25% on National Nosocomial Infection Survey [NNIS] levels for a similar patient population). We found that performance for each of these four process measures varied widely in our ICU and, while our performance on some measures was good, in only 30% of ventilator days did patients receive all four processes.

Fourth, we chose process measures that reflected changes we could make in our practice. It would have been illogical to focus on a measure that providers are unable to change. In other words, data management requires people management for success.

When selecting measures, we considered not only the clinical rationale of collecting data, but also the business rationale, necessitating knowledge of the costs of data collection and potential cost savings from improving performance. As such, we may not have wanted to focus on measuring performance if the cost of collecting the data exceeded the potential benefit from the improvement. This could be problematic when sophisticated risk adjustment methods require physiologic data that might be burdensome to collect in hospitals without automated data collection. In selecting our process measures, we felt that the potential benefit to our patients far exceeded any cost of data collection, especially given that we had an online clinical documentation system to support our efforts.

Finally, data do not improve patient care, people do. As such, it was imperative that the measures we chose were meaningful, scientifically sound, generalizable, and interpretable (McGlynn, 1998). To accomplish this, these measures were designed and implemented with the same rigor applied in clinical research. Process measures evaluate how we provide care, may be easier to measure and implement compared to outcome measures, and provide important insight into care (Pronovost et al., 2001). One of our process measures was the percent of patients on mechanical ventilation that have the head of the bed elevated at least 30 degrees. Process measures can be used to give immediate feedback to providers regarding their performance, allowing for rapid improvements in care. Outcome measures, like mortality, require longer periods of observation and, because events may be rare, feedback to providers takes longer. There are several additional important advantages of evaluating process measures—they generally have face validity for providers, meaning that providers often believe they can use the data to improve care, and risk adjustment is less important so broad implementation is feasible (Pronovost et al., 2001). Indeed, five out of the eight core measures selected by JCAHO for evaluating ICU quality and safety are process measures (www.jcaho.org).

What Changes Could We Make That Would Result in an Improvement?

One significant barrier to improving performance is that ICU care is a particularly complex and dynamic process. As such, it seems unlikely that one approach will be effective in all patient populations and all ICU settings, just as one measure will not provide a complete picture of quality. Indeed, strategies that combine different approaches are often more successful in changing performance than any single approach (Grol, 2001). Two strategies that have been successfully employed in the aviation industry to improve performance include interventions to reduce complexity and creating redundancies in the system to ensure that critical processes occur. (Institute of Medicine, 1999). To date, these strategies have not been fully evaluated in critical care.

Much of health care is delivered in complex processes. Because each step in a process has an independent probability of failure, care processes that require more steps are more likely to fail than processes that require fewer steps. In an earlier safety project, we found that there were 107 steps to administer medications in our ICU, from writing an order to giving the medication. Given this, the high rate of medication errors could be predicted. As experts in quality improvement say, "Every system is perfectly designed to achieve exactly the results it gets" (Berwick, 1996). To improve, we must change the systems, not individual providers. To decrease complexity, providers need to understand the system and reduce the number of steps in a process (Kenegy, Berwick, & Shore, 1999). In planning our safety improvement project, we needed to understand the system in which we provide care to mechanically ventilated patients, and to streamline our care processes to reflect the key evidence-based practices.

One approach to decrease complexity is to bundle care processes. A *care bundle* is a group or collection of process measures regarding a specific disease state that provides more robust insight into quality of care than any single measure. Based on the evidence, a ventilator bundle for patients requiring mechanical ventilation could include elevating the HOB, providing DVT and PUD prophylaxis, holding sedation, and assessing for readiness to extubate on a daily basis. Measuring performance on care bundles may also increase the likelihood of observing the anticipated impact on patient outcome if the evidence supports more than one care process. For example, we may not see an improvement in mortality for ventilated patients if patients always have the head of the bed elevated, yet providers fail to evaluate the ability to wean and extubate daily, or fail to titrate sedation such that the patient can follow commands at least once a day.

Another key concept used to improve safety in the aviation industry is independent redundancy; that is, if something is a critical step in a process, we can engage independent caregivers to ensure the process occurs. The use of checklists, for example, is an independent redundancy that is believed to have significantly improved safety in aviation and anesthesiology. (Institute of Medicine, 2001). Unfortunately, we have not fully applied the concept of independent redundancy in critical care.

Providers do not work in isolation. A team approach is imperative to create a culture of safety in which staff members are collectively committed to quality care. Crew resource management programs have been associated with improvements in the aviation industry (Helmreich & Merritt, 1998). Team training, based on the principles successfully used in aviation, may help to improve communication among providers, reduce the risk of patient injury, and improve patient care.

Plan

We sought to ensure that for 90% of ventilator days, patients received all four of the care processes, called a "ventilator bundle" (Berenholtz, Milanovich, et al., 2004). To accomplish this goal we implemented the following interventions:

1. Administering a questionnaire to identify barriers to compliance with the ventilator bundle

2. Implementing an educational intervention to improve compliance with the ventilator bundle

3. Implementing a checklist to be completed daily during ICU rounds to ask providers whether patients were receiving these therapies

Do

Nurses were generally not aware of the evidence supporting the use of these processes in mechanically ventilated patients. For example, when asked why they elevate a mechanically ventilated patient's HOB, over 90% of nurses stated that they do so because the physician ordered it. In addition, many nurses believed that the patient's HOB was elevated, yet when we measured the angle of the bed, it was less than 30 degrees. These results suggested that we might be able to improve compliance with these processes if we could increase provider awareness of the evidence and encourage them to advocate for quality and patient safety.

To create redundancy, we developed a standardized checklist, called the "Daily Goals" form to ask whether physicians wrote orders for head of bed elevation, PUD prophylaxis, DVT prophylaxis, and to hold sedation. The checklist was also used to explicitly outline the patient's plan of care for the day. The checklist was completed on all patients by the ICU resident or nurse practitioner during rounds, signed by the fellow or attending physician, and handed to the patient's nurse before moving on to the next patient.

Study

As a result of these three interventions, the percent of ventilator days where patients received all four care processes in the ventilator bundle increased from 30% to 96% ($p < 0.001$) (unpublished data). Our improvement in performance was sustained. One hundred percent of patients requiring mechanical ventilation received all four care processes 8 months after the start of our study. In addition, all providers interviewed reported that the format of the Daily Goals form was easy to understand and could be completed in less than 3 minutes.

Act

Because the Daily Goals form was so successful, the form is now routinely used in our ICU. In fact, several other ICUs within our organization have adopted the form, and plans are being made to spread to the remaining ICUs.

Conclusion

In our case discussion, we described how we developed an integrated approach to improving quality and safety in our ICU, coupled with the concepts of care bundles, independent redundancy, and reducing complexity to enhance provider compliance with the use of evidence-based therapies, and therefore improve quality and safety of care for patients requiring mechanical ventilation. Importantly, our approach is generalizable. Similar results have been observed in several other ICUs as part of a quality improvement collaborative supported by the IHI and VHA, Inc. (Pronovost et al., 2003). Additional areas that are ripe for measurement as a care bundle include care for the sepsis patient and efforts to minimize transfusion requirements.

References

Andrew, L. B., Stocking, C., Krizek, T., Gottlieb, L., Krizek, C., Vargish, T., et al. (1997). An alternative strategy for studying adverse drug events in medical care. *Lancet, 349*(9048), 309–313.

Angus, D. C., Kelley, M. A., Schmitz, R. J., White, A., Popovich, J., et al. (2000). Current and projected workshop requirements for the care of the critically ill patient and patients with pulmonary disease: Can we meet the requirements of an aging population? *Journal of the American Medical Association, 284,* 2762–2770.

Attia, J., Ray, J. G., Cook, D. L., Douketis, J., Ginsberg, J. S., & Geerts, W. H. (2001). Deep vein thrombosis in critically ill adults. *Archives of Internal Medicine, 161*(10), 1268–1279.

Azouley, E. et al. (2001). Meeting the needs of intensive care unit patient families: A multicenter study, *Critical Care Medicine, 163*(4), 135–139.

Berenholtz, S. M., Dorman, T., Ngo, K., & Pronovost, P. J. (2002). Qualitative review of intensive care unit quality indicators. *Journal of Critical Care, 17,* 1–12.

Berenholtz, S. M., Milanovich, S., Faircloth, A., Prow, D. T., Earsing, K., Lipsett, P., Dorman, T., Pronovost, P. J. (2004). Improving care for the ventilated patient. *Joint Commission Journal on Quality and Safety, 30*(4), 195–204.

Bernard, G. R., Vincent, J. L., LaRosa, S. P., Dhainaut, J. F., Lopez-Rodriguez, A, Steingrub, J. S., et al. (2001). Efficacy and safety of recombinant human activated protein C for severe sepsis. *New England Journal of Medicine, 344,* 699–709.

Bero, L. A., Grilli, R., Grimshaw, J. M., Harvey, E., Oxman, A. D., & Thomson, M. A. (2001). Closing the gap between research and practice: An overview of systematic reviews of interventions to promote the implementation of research findings. The Cochrane Effective Practice and Organization of Care Review Group. *British Medical Journal, 322,* 1258–1259.

Berwick, D. M. (1996). A primer on leading the improvement of systems. *British Medical Journal, 12,* 619–622.

Brook, A. D., Ahrens, T. S., Schaiff, R., Prentice, D., Sherman, G., Shannon, W., & Kollef, M. H. (1999). Effect of a nursing-implemented sedation protocol on the duration of mechanical ventilation. *Critical Care Medicine, 27,* 2609–2615.

Brook, R. H., McGlynn, E. A., & Cleary, P. D. (1996). Quality of health care. Part 2: Measuring quality of care. *New England Journal of Medicine, 335,* 966–970.

Cabana, M. D., Rand, C. S., Powe, N. R., Wu, A. W., Wilson, M. H., Abboud, P. A., & Rubin, H. R. (1999). Why don't physicians follow clinical practice guidelines? A framework for improvement. *Journal of the American Medical Association, 282,* 1458–1465.

Cook, D., Guyatt, G., Marshall, J., Leasa, D., Fuller, H., Hall, R., et al. (1998). A comparison of sucralfate and ranitidine for the prevention of upper gastrointestinal bleeding in patients requiring mechanical ventilation. Canadian Critical Care Trials Group. *New England Journal of Medicine, 338,* 791–797.

Cook, D. J., Meade, M. O., Hand, L. E., & McMullin, J. P. (2002). Toward understanding evidence uptake: Semirecumbency for pneumonia prevention. *Critical Care Medicine, 30,* 1272–1277.

Davis, D., O'Brien, M. A., Freemantle, N., Wolf, F. M., Mazmanian, P., & Taylor-Vaisey, A. (1999). Impact of formal continuing medical education: Do conferences, workshops, rounds, and other traditional continuing education activities change physician behavior or health care outcomes? *Journal of the American Medical Association, 282,* 867–874.

Donchin, Y., Gopher, D., Olin, M., Badihi, Y., Biesky, M., Sprung, C. L., et al. (1995). A look into the nature and causes of human errors in the intensive care unit. *Critical Care Medicine, 23,* 294–300.

Drakulovic, M. B., Torres, A., Bauer, T. T., Nicolas, J. M., Nogue, S., & Ferrer, M. (1999). Supine body position as a risk factor for nosocomial pneumonia in mechanically-ventilated patients: A randomized trial. *Lancet, 354,* 1851–1858.

Grol, R. (2001). Improving the quality of medical care: Building bridges among professional pride, payer profit, and patient satisfaction. *Journal of the American Medical Association, 286,* 2578–2585.

Grol, R., & Grimshaw, J. (1999). Evidence-based implementation of evidence-based medicine. *Joint Commission Journal of Quality Improvement, 25,* 506–513.

Halpern, N. A., Bettes, L., & Greenstein, R. (1994). Federal and nationwide intensive care units and healthcare costs: 1986–1992. *Critical Care Medicine, 22,* 2001–2007.

Helmreich, R. L., & Merritt, A. C. (1998). *Culture at work in aviation and medicine: National, organizational, and professional influences.* Aldershot, Hampshire, United Kingdom:Ashgate.

Heyland, D. K., Tranmer, J. E., & Kingston General Hospital ICU Research Working Group. (2001). Measuring family satisfaction with care in the intensive care unit: The development of a questionnaire and preliminary results. *Journal of Critical Care, 16,* 142–149.

Institute of Medicine. (1999). *To Err Is Human: Building a Safer Health System.* Washington, DC: National Academy Press.

Institute of Medicine. (2001). *Crossing the Quality Chasm: A New Health System for the 21st Century.* Washington, DC: National Academy Press.

Kenegy, J. W., Berwick, D. M., & Shore, M. F. (1999). Service quality in health care. *Journal of the American Medical Association, 281,* 661–665.

Kollef, M. H. (1999). The prevention of ventilator-associated pneumonia. *New England Journal of Medicine, 340,* 627–634.

Kress, J. P., Pohlman, A. S., O'Connor, M. F., & Hall, J. B. (2000). Daily interruption of sedative infusions in critically ill patients undergoing mechanical ventilation. *New England Journal of Medicine, 342,* 1471–1477.

Leape, L. L., Cullen, D. J., Clapp, M. D., Burdick, E., Demonaco, H. J., Erickson, J. I., & Bates, D. W. (1999). Pharmacist participation on physician rounds and adverse drug events in the intensive care unit. *Journal of the American Medical Association, 282,* 267–270.

Marelich, G. P., Murin, S., Battistella, F., Inciardi, J., Vierra, T., & Roby, M. (2000). Protocol weaning of mechanical ventilation in medical and surgical patients by respiratory care practitioners and nurses: Effect on weaning time and incidence of ventilator-associated pneumonia. *Chest, 118,* 459–467.

McGlynn, E. A. (1998). Choosing and evaluating clinical performance measures. *Joint Commission Journal on Quality Improvement, 24,* 470–479.

McGlynn, E. A., & Asch, S. M. (1998). Developing a clinical performance measure. *American Journal of Preventive Medicine, 14*(3 Suppl), 14–21.

Pronovost, P. J., Berenholtz, S. M., Ngo, K., McDowell, M., Holzmueller, C., Haraden, C., Resar, R., Rainey, T., Nolan, T., Dorman, T. (2003). Developing and pilot testing quality indicators in the intensive care unit. *Journal of Critical Care, 18*(3), 145–155.

Pronovost, P. J., Berenholtz, S., Dorman, T., Lipsett, P. A., Simmonds, T., & Haraden, C. (2003). Improving communication in the ICU using daily goals. *Journal of Critical Care, 18*(2), 71–75.

Pronovost, P. J., Dang, D., Dorman, T., Lipsett, P. A., Garrett, E., Jenckes, M., & Bass, E. B. (2001). Intensive care unit nurse staffing and the risk for complications after abdominal aortic surgery. *Effective Clinical Practice, 4,* 199–206.

Pronovost, P. J., Miller, M. R., Dorman, T., Berenholtz, S. M., & Rubin, H. (2001). Developing and implementing measures of quality of care in the intensive care unit. *Current Opinion in Critical Care, 7,* 297–303.

Rubin, H. R., Pronovost, P., & Diette, G. B. (2001). From a process of care to a measure: The development and testing of a quality indicator. *International Journal of Quality Health Care, 13,* 489–496.

Sackett, D. L., Rosenberg, W. M., Gray, J. A., Haynes, R. B., & Richardson, W. S. (1996). Evidence based medicine: What it is and what it isn't. *British Medical Journal, 312,* 71–72.

van den Berghe, G., Wouters, P., Weekers, F., Verwaest, C., Bruyninckx, F., Schetz, M., et al. (2001). Intensive insulin therapy in the critically ill patients. *New England Journal of Medicine, 345,* 1359–1367.

Wasser, T., Pasquale, M. A., Matchett, S. C., Bryan, Y., & Pasquale, M. (2001). Establishing reliability and validity of the critical care family satisfaction survey. *Critical Care Medicine, 29,* 192–196.

Zimmerman, J. E., Wagner, D. P., Draper, E. A., Wright, L., Alzola, C., & Knaus, W. A. (1998). Evaluation of acute physiology and chronic health evaluation III: Predictions of hospital mortality in an independent database. *Critical Care Medicine, 26,* 1317–1326.

CHAPTER 8

Medication Reconciliation in the ICU

Rhonda Wyskiel, RN, BSN*

Mandalyn Schwarz, RN*

M s. W is back in the ICU again. She had been on amiodarone at home, as well as during her ICU stay for chronic atrial fibrillation. She was discharged to the floor 2 days ago, but is now readmitted in atrial fibrillation with rapid ventricular response. The ICU nurse received the transfer report. Initially on transfer to the floor, her amiodarone had not been ordered. The team wondered if receiving the medication would have prevented her readmission. The performance improvement team had studied patients that were readmitted to the unit, but had never discussed transfer orders as a potential problem.

Background

While attending a medication safety lecture at an Institute for Healthcare Improvement (IHI) workshop in June 2000, the opportunity to improve safety within the Weinberg Intensive Care Unit (ICU) emerged. The safety opportunity was the reconciliation of prehospital medications. Reconciliation first involves a comparison of a patient's prehospital medications and newly prescribed medications, and then a comparison of the prehospital and newly prescribed medications to those ordered on transfer orders for accuracy. This is an example of the concept of *independent redundancy*. This measure had not been evaluated as part of performance improvement in our new 14-bed ICU.

*The Johns Hopkins Hospital

This chapter will describe the results of our pilot study, and the redesigned work process. This project and the implementation of this new process have now ingrained medication safety into our routine and standard of care, and has resulted in a reduction of transfer medication inaccuracy to essentially no medication errors on transfer. We will discuss barriers to this change process along with lessons learned during the journey.

Plan

Two nurses collected data to determine the scope of the problem. The nurses summarized the transferring patient's prehospital medications and newly prescribed medications, and then compared the list to the transfer orders for accuracy. The team reviewed inaccuracies in drugs, dosages, routes, and frequencies. A medication reconciliation form, also known as the discharge survey, was developed to measure and improve the number of potential medication errors.

Twenty-four charts were selected randomly as patients were discharged from the ICU. Out of 20 charts that were audited, 30 potential medication errors were discovered. All were corrected on detection by calling the transferring physician and clarifying the medications ordered or omitted. The potential adverse drug events included wrong allergies or none documented at all, discrepancies in already standing ICU orders, and omission in returning a patient to his or her prehospital medications. The errors included medications such as sedatives, beta-blockers, antihypertensives, cardiac medications, pulmonary medications, synthroid, antibiotics, and GI prophylaxis. These findings were so surprising that the staff realized that there was an immediate and urgent need for an improved work process.

Do

Because of the large number of preventable medication errors, the medication reconciliation process and form needed to become part of our admission and discharge process. Staff education was initiated immediately, with discussion of results of the pilot and details of how to complete the discharge survey and follow up with transferring physicians. Nurses received education on communication techniques to enhance problem solving when they called transferring physicians to discuss differences in the reconciliation of medication orders.

Study

Over a 6-month period, reconciliation of medication demonstrated improvements. Data included compliance, the actual number of medication orders changed (comparing this at the patient level and at the medication level), and the accuracy of staff compliance in filling out the data collection form. The information was presented to the hospital safety committee, various management committees, various nursing and departmental performance improvement committees, and other nursing units that were interested in replicating the study.

Act

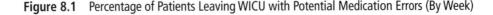

Medication reconciliation became part of the standard of care in the WICU. However, numerous PDSA cycles were required to make medication reconciliation an independent redundancy in the WICU. Figure 8.1 illustrates the reduction in the percentage of patients leaving the WICU with medication errors by week. The baseline data can be viewed at weeks one and three, demonstrating a 94% medication error rate for patients transferred from the WICU. After initiation of the medication reconciliation process, the percentage of patients with potential medication error was decreased to 50%, and then to 0%. The increase between weeks 13 and 17 showed the need for continued education and staff support.

Figure 8.1 Percentage of Patients Leaving WICU with Potential Medication Errors (By Week)

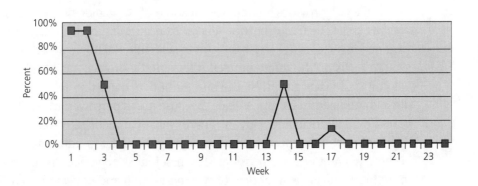

Figure 8.2 demonstrates the decrease in the medication reconciliation intervention rate over 2 years. The calculation used to determine the intervention rate was the number of orders changed on transfer orders in response to the reconciliation process divided by the number of total orders; the premeasures and postmeasures for the study remained the same. If a medication discrepancy was found on a transfer order, the order was changed by the physician, and then counted as a potential medication error.

Since the implementation of the medication reconciliation process, potential medication errors on transfer have been significantly reduced. Nurses continue to intervene by using the medication reconciliation tool on 35% of our patients, demonstrating improvement, but the need for continued work.

Figure 8.2 Medication Reconciliation Intervention Rate Over 2 Years

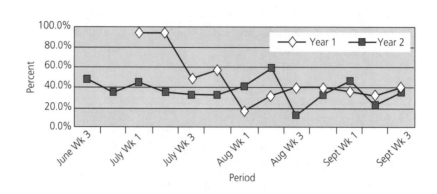

Lessons Learned

Medication reconciliation has increased communication and teamwork among the ICU staff team members and physicians. It has allowed us to improve the safety of our patients during the "hand-off" of care from the ICU setting to the floor setting, improving safety and continuity for patients. This project has also encouraged us as a team to include both patients and families in their care, promoting collaboration between hospital staff and patient.

Table 8.1 provides a summary of some of the major barriers overcome in this process. The major barrier related to time. With high acuity, patient flow, and nursing vacancies, it was difficult to schedule RN hours away from the bedside to focus on the safety project. Although the project was a high priority for all unit staff (MDs and RNs), the burden of data collection fell on the RNs, and the clinical needs took precedence. Because it was perceived as additional work, it was difficult to achieve buy-in. There was no immediate reward for the work input of reviewing the chart and collecting the data. In addition, the data collection tool required five revisions. The first four were very detailed and not user friendly, requiring a great deal of communication and education to make them usable. Coupled with the normal resistance to any change, this made the process difficult. We had trouble communicating quickly enough, and translating the data into information that was usable for the staff. The project coordinators realized that they needed a variety of additional skills in metrics, data management, and graphic display of results. Results needed to be displayed appropriately and in a timely manner to keep the focus and attention of the staff on the safety priority. There were struggles with interdisciplinary collaboration (RNs and MDs) when RNs called MDs to validate order accuracy. Although the project was public, the MDs questioned the reasoning behind the new validation system and additional calls. It was difficult to refocus from the burden of the call to a common goal of patient safety. We needed to partner with a physician leader in the safety effort to reinforce the process and support the nurses.

Table 8.1 Barriers and Success Strategies

Barrier	Description of Barrier	Strategies for Success
Time	Conflict to schedule RN hours away from the bedside to do safety work. Difficult to achieve buy-in. Time consuming process.	Constant refocus on priority Managerial support
Data collection	RNs required a large amount of education to perform data collection, tracking, and data analysis.	Revisions to data collection tool to reduce burden and create independent redundancies
Resistance to change	RNs and MDs resisted increased workload of project.	Displaying dramatic results and responding to suggestions
Communication	There was poor communication and dissemination of study results with the RNs and physicians in the unit who were helping with data collection.	Skill building in metrics, data collection and analysis, and graphic display of improvements
Collaboration	Interdisciplinary collaboration (RNs and MDs) was a struggle.	Commitment to patient safety Physician and nursing leader support Focusing on a common goal: patient safety

Table 8.2 summarizes some of our most important lessons learned. First, when the urgency of the results are understood by the team, commitment follows. Conveying this urgency requires attention to communication and presentation of results through formal and informal channels. Also, when planning a safety project, consider time and resources in the plan to ensure that project outcomes will be met. The unit staff and physicians are the team that together will make the difference in patient safety. Achieving their buy-in up front and individualizing the plan for each unit, is the most important factor to the success of a reconciliation project. It promotes a smooth change process, improves compliance with data reporting, and helps them to understand the impact of their actions.

Safety teams may need to seek resources to gain skills for accurate and reliable data collection and presentation. This is important because data drives change—when the team sees the data, there is an innate responsibility to act on it. Work processes will also need to change; for example, providing physicians with comprehensive medication discharge information in a standard place is a timely and efficient means to improve transfer order accuracy.

The documentation was time consuming and added more responsibility to the nurses. Initially, staff said the process was a burden, but then it slowly became incorporated into their routine. It resulted in a new work process that prioritizes patient safety. It also broadened the nurses' knowledge base regarding each individual patient, providing them a safe, smooth course of care.

Table 8.2 Lessons Learned

1. When the urgency of the results are understood by the team, commitment follows.
2. To accomplish improvements in a safety initiative, time and resources need to be planned.
3. Achieving staff buy-in up front promotes a smooth change process and improves compliance with data reporting.
4. Resources are needed to gain skills for accurate and reliable data collection.
5. Data drives change and must be included in any change process.
6. Providing physicians with comprehensive medication discharge information in a standard place is a timely and efficient means to improve transfer order accuracy.
7. When participation, accountability, and recognition are shared, they result in increased team ownership in safety initiatives.

Conclusion

In conclusion, this is not a project, but a process—a new way of thinking in the ICU. Our project demonstrates the urgent need for medication reconciliation in the ICU. Our discovery of the magnitude of the problem, and the improvements demonstrated through this project, lead us to believe that medication reconciliation should become a part of a standard ICU metric for safety improvements. This will necessitate a critical examination of current work processes required, nurse and physician collaboration, and a mutual focus on patient safety.

CHAPTER 9

Chemotherapy Safety

MiKaela Olsen RN, MS, OCN*

It was a typical day in a busy oncology infusion area. Many patients were expected, and the nurses began to prepare for the day. Preprinted chemotherapy orders were being utilized in order to decrease errors associated with illegible handwritten orders. The orders prompted the physician to write down the patient-specific data such as pertinent lab values, height, weight, and allergies. Mrs. Jones arrived for her chemotherapy, which had already been prepared by the pharmacy. The nurses checked the chemotherapy orders and calculations and began to prepare for the administration of Mrs. Jones's chemotherapy. The pertinent lab value in this case was the creatinine, as the chemotherapy drug was very nephrotoxic. The physician had written a creatinine of 0.9 mg/dl on the preprinted orders. The nurse noted the creatinine that the physician had reported, and proceeded with the chemotherapy. Several days after chemotherapy Mrs. Jones was admitted to the hospital after presenting in an emergency room with bleeding, oliguria, neutropenia, and severe fatigue. Her creatinine was noted to be 8.7 mg/dl in the emergency room. Upon further review it was discovered that the creatinine that the physician documented on the preprinted orders was over a month old, and that the most recent creatinine, at the time chemotherapy was given, was actually 7.0 mg/dl. This example underscores the importance of independent validation of each required safety check and the data used to determine chemotherapy eligibility. In this case, the pharmacists and nurses involved should have independently verified pertinent lab values from an original source prior to dispensing and administering the chemotherapy.

*Oncology & BMT Clinical Nurse Specialist
Sidney Kimmel Comprehensive Cancer Center at the Johns Hopkins Hospital

Background

Providing care for the cancer patient utilizing chemotherapeutic agents is a high-risk process, involving multiple providers. Catastrophic patient injury and deaths have been linked to errors in the processes related to chemotherapy. The term *chemotherapy process* includes prescribing, dispensing, and administering. The academic research environment presents a unique challenge because of our complex patient population. At the Sidney Kimmel Comprehensive Cancer Center (SKCCC) located in the Johns Hopkins Hospital, more than 70 chemotherapeutic agents are administered as both standard and research treatment plans. Drug development and phase I studies are another cornerstone of our National Cancer Institute (NCI)–designated comprehensive cancer center. This chemotherapy-diverse environment challenges the clinician's ability to maintain expertise. With less experienced staff and an increasing clinical treatment complexity, chemotherapy errors have become problematic. In addition, the institutional policies and procedures regarding chemotherapy are lengthy and complicated, making it difficult for staff to remember all of the required checks and to complete these checks in a consistent manner.

A number of sentinel events occurred related to chemotherapy between 1999 and 2000, each prompting a root cause analysis and performance improvement initiatives. Contributing to errors were inconsistent practices related to prescribing, dispensing, and administering chemotherapy. The outcome of these initiatives included a revised Johns Hopkins Hospital (JHH) Chemotherapy Policy; the institution of new safety requirements (e.g., double-checks at each step in the process, verification of all pertinent laboratory values); the addition of a chemotherapy treatment note; the creation of a prechemotherapy administration checklist; the establishment of a comprehensive outpatient treatment chart; and the development of standard, preprinted chemotherapy orders. Monthly multidisciplinary updates and discussions were conducted to include all chemotherapy errors. This chapter will review the chemotherapy safety initiatives that were designed and implemented using the Plan-Do-Study-Act process in order to decrease chemotherapy errors.

Plan

In preparation for the project, a team was formed to review the current policy requirements, current practice, and previous chemotherapy errors. This oncology team consisted of a physician, a pharmacist, a nurse manager, and a clinical nurse specialist. The team goals included:

1. Revision of the chemotherapy policy
2. Development of checklists to aid in the compliance and accuracy of safety checks

3. Implementation of an online medication error reporting system

4. Staff education regarding the importance of near-miss reporting

5. Development of preprinted chemotherapy orders for disease-based regimens

6. Development of pharmacy and nursing drug-specific chemotherapy guidelines

7. Development of a patient-specific treatment plan for all patients receiving chemotherapy

8. Development of an outpatient treatment chart to house chemotherapy orders and notes

9. Development of an *Oncology Clinical Tools Icon,* which provided direct access to the policies and procedures, research protocols, medication error reporting systems, and other tools used frequently by oncology providers

Do

The team began their work with the revision of the multidisciplinary, institution-wide chemotherapy policy, which became the foundation for the safety projects that followed. During the policy review it became apparent that the extensive safety checks required were cumbersome and difficult to carry out in a consistent manner. The team recognized that the current chemotherapy process was inconsistently understood and applied among all disciplines, which placed all providers at high risk for chemotherapy errors. Using the operating room checklist as a model, chemotherapy dispensing and administering checklists were developed and piloted. The checklists contained the mandatory safety checks, all of which were specified in the protocol requirements, to aid the pharmacy and nursing personnel when dispensing and administering chemotherapy (see Figure 9.1). Hospital-wide education was completed, and the chemotherapy administration checklist was implemented. The administration checklist became a requirement for every dose of chemotherapy and biotherapy administered hospital-wide for oncology and nononcology patients.

In reviewing near-miss error reporting data, the team recognized that the percentage of chemotherapy errors reported, that did not reach the patient, was low. The online medication error reporting system was piloted on one oncology unit and then rolled out center-wide. Extensive multidisciplinary education was completed to develop a culture that fostered a nonpunative environment and stressed the importance of near-miss reporting. The implementation of this system increased near-miss reporting in the oncology center significantly (see Figure 9.2). The team reviewed all actual and near-miss data in an effort to analyze and

Figure 9.1 Chemotherapy Administration Checklist

THE JOHNS HOPKINS HOSPITAL Chemotherapy Administration CHECKLIST			For addressograph plate		
SIGNATURE/TITLE		INITIALS			

Date:	Regimen:	Order #:	Allergies: ☐ Yes ☐ No List:_____			
Central line present for continuous IV vesicant chemo **Yes** **Blood return present** **N/A**			Weight: Kg	Height: cm/inches	BSA	IBW

CHECKLIST	INTITIALS	Comments:
BEFORE ADMINISTRATION OF THE _FIRST_ DOSE OF EACH CHEMOTHERAPY AGENT ORDERED:		
1. Order includes any supportive care medications (e.g., Premeds, antiemetics, hydration, growth factors, emerg. meds etc.).		None required per regimen ☐
2. Confirm presence of consent (if applicable).		* Must be located in the medical records
3. Patient, family, and/or caregiver have received written or verbal education.		
4. Patient understands the treatment plan, toxicities, and side effects and wishes to proceed.		
BEFORE _EVERY_ DOSE OF A CHEMOTHERAPY AGENT: **(Practitioner administering chemo)**		
1. Doses are acceptable based on: (refer to policy for definitions) ☐ Standard ☐ JCCI Research ☐ Individual protocol therapy *Web address for oncology center research protocols: JHMCIS.JHMI.edu/oncres		Reference for dosing of individual chemotherapy is placed in chart. ☐ If a reference doesn't exist for individual chemotherapy _two attending physicians_ have signed the treatment plan. ☐
2. Treatment note/Pediatric roadmap includes: Date, indication for chemo, chemo agents used, doses, schedule, dose modification and rationale for modifications (if applicable). *For standard regimens e.g. VAD, CHOP, JHH Oncology preprinted chemo orders doses do not need to be rewritten in note, unless modified.*		* Do not administer chemo without attending co-signature on chemo orders and treatment note/pediatric roadmap.
3. Treatment note/Pediatric roadmap is written or co-signed by attending physician.		
4. If on research protocol: note includes protocol #, arm, and cycle or phase.		N/A ☐
5. Lab values that would modify administration of chemo are WNL (labs should be within 7 days unless otherwise specified) * acceptable values are based on protocol requirements or dept. standards.		Order received to hold chemo. ☐ Order received to proceed. ☐
6. Assess patient's prior tolerance to chemo and note any existing side effects or toxicities; notify physician if indicated.		
7. Correct drug, dose, route, patient name, history number, birthdate, and patient ID band (JHH Medical ID card in outpatient areas) verified with patient and chemo orders at bedside/chair.		
VAILDATION BEFORE _EVERY_ DOSE OF A CHEMOTHERAPY AGENT: **(2 practioners independently check)**		*** Document on pg 2 of chemo checklist**
1. Chemo orders are written or co-signed by attending physician.		* Do not proceed without attending signature.
2. MD orders contain drug, dose, (e.g., units/m² or units/kg), dosing interval, duration of therapy, dilutent type, and volume and rate (if applicable), Ht, Wt, & BSA.		N/A (prescribed dose for nononcology patient where dose is not used for dosing) ☐ * Only abbreviations on Appendix A of MDU001 are acceptable.
3. Multi-day continuous infusion chemo includes total daily dose and total multi-day hours of infusion.		N/A ☐
4. Doses based on renal function, ideal or adjusted Wt., or other formulas include calculations.		

© The Johns Hopkins Hospital

Figure 9.2 Total Near-Miss Errors Reported (Online Error Reporting System Initiated FY02) SKCCC at the Johns Hopkins Hospital

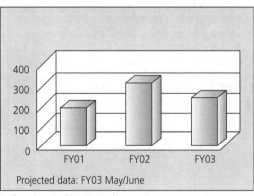

Projected data: FY03 May/June

© The Johns Hopkins Hospital

prevent future chemotherapy errors. Multidisciplinary medication error review conferences were established to provide a forum for the discussion of errors and prevention strategies.

After analyzing the literature and previous chemotherapy errors it became apparent that the use of handwritten physician chemotherapy orders was a high-risk practice. Many clarifications were required following the receipt of handwritten orders from the physician. These clarifications were often related to missing patient-specific data elements, as well as incomplete supportive care orders (e.g., antiemetic not ordered for a highly emetogenic regimen). Pharmacy and nursing time was compromised when multiple clarifications were required. In addition, regimens were often written inconsistently and thus administered inconsistently, which led to confusion among staff and patients. This knowledge, coupled with the impending initiation of a physician order entry system, became the impetus for the development of preprinted standard chemotherapy order sets. The SKCCC obtained a grant from MCIC Vermont, Inc. to assist with funding for the development of these orders. An additional inpatient/outpatient team was formed that included physicians, pharmacists, nurse managers, clinical nurse specialists, and nurse clinicians working directly at the bedside. This team designed, reviewed, and implemented the standard preprinted orders for use with chemotherapy. These orders contained all necessary information (e.g., prechemotherapy test results such as creatinine clearance, current lab values, cumulative doses, dose modification rationale) and supportive care requirements that should be linked to specific chemotherapy medications (see Figure 9.3). The multidisciplinary approach to the development of these orders helped to ensure that they were organized, clear, and understandable to all. Today over 100 preprinted chemotherapy orders have

Figure 9.3   A Preprinted Chemotherapy Order

THE JOHNS HOPKINS HOSPITAL
ORDER SHEET
CHOP for Non Hodgkin's Lymphoma
Cyclophosphamide/Doxorubicin/Vincristine/Prednisone
(Standard Chemotherapy Orders)   *For addressograph plate*

Page _____   (Page 1 Of 2)

Ordered		SIGN EACH ENTRY – INCLUDE ID NUMBER *use a ball point pen, press firmly*	Noted by	Order completed		Initials
Date	Time			Date	Time	
		00 Ht:_____cm, Wt:_____kg, BSA:_____m^2				
		01 Cycle #_____ Day 1: (_____/_____/____)				
		02 • **Treatment Note is:** ❑ Attached (outpatient) OR in medical record (inpatient) ❑ In OCIS ❑ In EPR date (_____/_____/____)				
		03 • **Notify Attending MD** Abs. Neutr. Ct. (ANC) < 1,000/mm^3 Plt < 100,000/mm^3 Bilirubin ≥ 2 mg/dl SCr ≥ 2 mg/dl Note: Counts must have been drawn within 3 days of giving chemotherapy.				
		04 • **Hydration** (Pre-cyclophosphamide) IV fluids _____				
		05 • **Premedication** Dolasetron 100 mg p.o. 30 minutes prior to chemo on Day 1.				
		06 **Prochlorperazine** 10 mg p.o. every 4 hours p.r.n. for nausea/vomiting.				
		07 • **Chemotherapy** Doxorubicin 50 mg/m^2 = _____ mg IV Push on day 1. ❑ Dose modification reason _____ **Modified doxorubicin dose** _____mg/m^2 =_____mg IV Push on Day 1. (Patient's cumulative lifetime anthracycline dose including this dose = _____ mg/m^2) Anthracycline medication name _____ doses=_____mg/m2 Anthracycline medication name _____ doses=_____mg/m2 Anthracycline medication name _____ doses=_____mg/m2				
		08 **Vincristine** 1.4mg/m^2 = _____ mg IV Push on Day 1. **Note: Maximum dose is 2mg.** ❑ Dose modification reason _____ **Modified vincristine dose** _____mg/m^2 =_____mg IV Push on Day 1.				
		09 **Cyclophosphamide** 750 mg/m^2 = _____mg IV in 250 ml D5W over one hour on Day 1. ❑ Dose modification reason _____ **Modified cyclophosphamide dose** _____mg/m^2 =_____mg IV in 250 ml D5W over one hour on Day 1.				
		10 _____ MD, _____ ID # _____ Beeper				
		11 _____ Attending MD, _____ ID# _____ Beeper				
		12 (Continued on page 2)				

❑ Order is faxed or sent to the pharmacy

Form #JHH-15-193060 (9/96)   Suffix #:
© The Johns Hopkins Hospital

been developed. In the future these orders will greatly assist in the initiation of a physician order entry system with disease-specific order sets.

The chemotherapy policy-required safety checks included many drug-specific parameters such as cumulative dosing guidelines, specific laboratory values that would preclude administration, dilution and mixing guidelines, and administration specifics. The nurse and pharmacy were not always in agreement about these drug-specific parameters and were often utilizing different references to obtain information. Joint nurse and pharmacy administration guidelines were developed by a clinical nurse specialist and then reviewed by nursing and pharmacy for final approval. These guidelines (see Figure 9.4) assist pharmacists and nurses in becoming familiar with specific chemotherapeutic/biologic agents and assist with consistent dispensing and administration of these medications. These guidelines will be available online for use hospital-wide.

One important safety requirement of the new chemotherapy policy included an attending physician treatment plan, to assist the nurse and pharmacists in verifying that the chemotherapy is appropriate for a specific patient. The treatment plan includes patient name, history number, indication for treatment, regimen, doses, specific cycle, phase, arm (if applicable), and length of therapy. Types of chemotherapy/biotherapy orders were further labeled as one of the following: standard, research, individual with a reference, and individual without a reference. The labeling of the types of chemotherapy/biotherapy assisted in providing a common nomenclature to guide providers in the determination of appropriate dosing. The four types of chemotherapy/biotherapy orders were defined as follows: 1) standard chemotherapy orders (as defined by SKCCC preprinted standard orders and/or an identified national standard of care regimen; 2) research protocol chemotherapy orders; 3) individual chemotherapy orders with a reference; 4) individual chemotherapy orders without a reference. The requirement for a reference was established to assist providers in the verification of appropriate dosing. In the absence of a reference, for individual therapy, an additional attending physician is required for verification of appropriateness of orders. The treatment note serves as a valuable tool for ensuring the described plan is for a specific patient. The requirements for a reference and treatment plan are included in the specific safety checks completed by all members of the chemotherapy process.

The treatment plan, orders, and reference must coexist in the chart so that all providers have immediate access to complete the required safety checks. The volume of outpatients seen daily in the oncology department made the availability of these documents in the chart an immense challenge. An outpatient oncology treatment chart that would be assembled the day prior to chemotherapy appointment dates was developed. The orders and treatment plans were assembled and verified in this chart the day prior so that nurses caring for patients on the day of the infusions would have direct access to this information without slowing down the process. By having the necessary components of the oncology medical record readily available, compliance in completing the required safety checks increased.

Figure 9.4 Nursing Chemotherapy Administration Guideline

Drug Mechanisms/ Indications	Common Doses	Administration	Side Effects/Toxicities	Nursing Considerations
Adriamycin (Doxorubicin hydrochloride/ Adria) *Anthracycline Antitumor Antibiotic* cell cycle non-specific Metabolized in the liver excreted mainly in bile and some in urine. Used in a variety of malignancies to include; Breast cancer, leukemia, soft tissue and bone sarcomas, multiple myeloma, SC lung cancer, bladder cancer, Hodgkin's disease, NHL, ovarian cancer, and more.	*Example:* 60–90 mg/m^2 IV bolus Q 3 weeks in individual therapy, 45–60 mg/m^2 IV Q 3 weeks in combination therapy or CIV over 3–4 days. Maximal lifetime dose = 550 mg/m^2 to prevent cardiac toxicity. Patients with previous mantle/chest radiation or cardiac dysfunction require dose adjustments (440 mg/m^2).	**VESICANT*** Administer IV preferably through a CVC. Use an infusion pump for all continuous infusions through a central line. If no CVC, administer peripherally using the IVSA technique. **Pertinent labs to check prior to administration:** Call MD if labs are not WNL-CBC, ANC >1000, plt >100 SGOT, SGPT, Alk. Phosp., Tbili, BUN, creatinine. Baseline ECG should be done. MUGA scan may be done prior to first dose. Assess concurrent cardiac risk factors. **Antidote for adriamycin—use cold and elevation, follow vesicant protocol for DMSO usage.**	**Hematologic:** Neutropenia is the dose-limiting toxicity, nadir 10–14 days. Recovery by day 21. Thrombocytopenia and anemia can also occur. **GI:** N/V—mod to severe emetogenicity. antiemetics required. Usually occurs within 1–3 hours of administration and can last 12–24 hours. Diarrhea can occur. Stomatitis is more common with higher doses and CIV infusions. **Cardiac:** Arrythmias, ECG changes, cardiomyopathy with subsequent CHF when doses exceed maximum lifetime allowance. Risk factors are prior mediastinal XRT, increasing age, and pre-existing cardiac disease. **Alopecia:** Usually total and reversible, occurs usually 5 weeks after initial treatment. Re-growth approx 3 months after completion. **Dermatologic:** *Hypersensitivity reactions along vein during administration. "Flare reaction." Hyperpigmentation of nail beds, radiation recall reactions. **Other:** Red/pink discoloration of urine; immediate onset, lasts X 1–2 days.	1. Instruct the patient on adriamycin administration and side effects. 2. Provide the patient with educational materials as appropriate. 3. Instruct the patient on signs and symptoms of infection, anemia, and thrombocytopenia and ways to prevent complications. 4. Assess previous radiation sites for recall reactions. Assess and tabulate total adriamycin patient has received. 5. Incompatible with many drugs so always verify compatibility. Incompatible with heparin and lasix.

The final step in the safety project was to ensure all oncology providers had easy access to online resources. With the advent of computerized databases and online department-wide policies and procedures, many providers were discouraged by their inability to quickly locate resources. A department-wide icon called the *Oncology Clinical Tools Icon* was developed, and was made available on all computers in the oncology department; to date it has had over 50,000 visitors (see Figure 9.5). The icon contains multiple links to various intranet and Internet sites used frequently by the oncology provider. In addition to links to online chemotherapy compatibility charts, drug information sheets, patient teaching materials, and policies and procedures, this icon provides direct access to all current research protocols and standard preprinted chemotherapy order sets, which can be printed instantly.

Study

In our institution the traditional primary measure for evaluation of chemotherapy errors has been the number of actual and near-miss errors in relation to the number of chemotherapy doses dispensed. This assumes all errors are reported, which, historically, has been a challenge. After initiating these tools, the SKCCC continued to evaluate all errors reported. The number of near-miss errors reported increased significantly for the first two fiscal years after the implementation of the online error reporting system and staff education; however, the number of significant errors has decreased since the initiation of the described safety measures. The recent decrease in near-miss reporting is thought to be related to a need for ongoing reinforcement and education regarding the importance of this type of reporting. Education targeted to all existing and new staff has been put into place to address these ongoing needs.

Act

Since implementation of the safety initiatives, few significant errors have occurred; however, the reported errors that have surfaced were unanticipated given the current safety checks and requirements. The system in which we operate continues to be fallible. Ongoing review of errors and intensive review of the system are absolute requirements. Three additional changes are actively being initiated: a chemotherapy survey tool, increased staff education, and a chemotherapy process review called Failure Modes Effects Analysis (FMEA).

The current dependence upon providers to report every near miss is incomplete, primarily due to lack of time. Providers continue to fix and mend potential errors before they reach the patient, but fail to report this "fix." This leaves all providers and patients vulnerable. In an attempt to collect more accurate error data, a chemotherapy survey tool was developed. This computerized data collection system is designed to assist a provider in auditing chemotherapy charts to determine if policy and procedures were followed; to determine if potential errors existed within chemotherapy orders, which were subsequently discovered by providers; and to collect more specific measures related

Figure 9.5   The *Oncology Clinical Tools Icon*

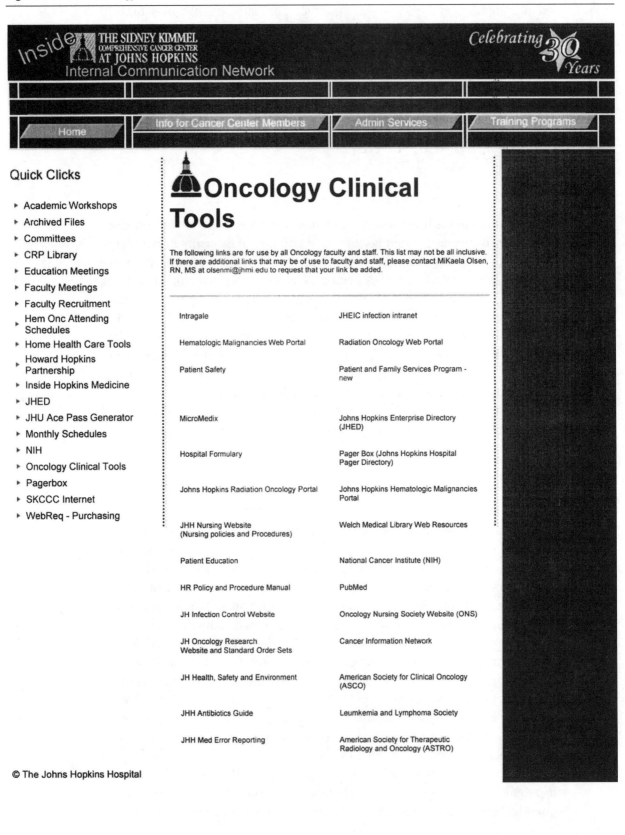

to the chemotherapy process that could assist in improving outcomes. The audit tool is located on all computers hospital-wide and uses an instant messaging function to submit data to a central database for analysis. In addition to current reported error data collection, the development of this audit tool will assist with necessary systems analysis and change.

Staff education regarding this complex process continues to be a challenge at our institution. All nurses complete the Oncology Nursing Society's Chemotherapy and Biotherapy Course and are required to attend annual chemotherapy competencies. Challenges continue to exist related to physician and pharmacy education regarding this process.

In an attempt to proactively identify potential errors in the system, the FMEA chemotherapy process is now part of our safety culture. "FMEA is a team-based, systematic, and proactive approach for identifying the ways that a process or design can fail, why it might fail, and how it can be made safer" (Joint Commission Resources, 2004, p. 15). The FMEA describes in detail the prescribing, dispensing, and administering process for chemotherapy. This process is likely to provide valuable insight into this complex process and strategies for preventing future errors.

Conclusion

In recent years the field of oncology has seen a dramatic rise in the number of new drugs available to cancer patients with various diseases. Many new classes of chemotherapy and biotherapy agents, as well as new combinations of treatment modalities, are emerging. The toxicity profiles are different and complicated. These issues present a great safety challenge to providers who prescribe, dispense, and administer these drugs to oncology patients. The work that our institution accomplished has been invaluable in assisting with the prevention of chemotherapy errors; however, this is an ongoing project that will need to exist for as long as we treat oncology patients. New chemotherapy and biotherapy safety challenges will emerge, and our institution is committed to working diligently to anticipate, prevent, and minimize harm to our patients.

Reference

Joint Commission Resources (2004, January). *Joint Commission Perspectives, 24*(1), p. 15. Available online at: http://www.jcaho.org/accredited+organizations/svnp/jcp-2004-january.pdf Accessed 06/30/04.

CHAPTER 10

Preventing Patient Aggression: Assessment and Reporting as First Steps

Karin Taylor, APRN, PMH*

Donna Brannan, RN, MSN**

Judith M. Rohde, RN, MS†

Gary Dunn, RN, MAS, MSN††

Bernard Vincent Keenan, RN, BC, MSN#

Geetha Jayaram, MD, MBA##

During an evening shift on a busy 22-bed psychiatric unit, a staff member was hit several times in the face by a patient. The unit was in an uproar; patients witnessed the assault, it took several staff members to restrain the patient, and the nurse was treated in the ED with subsequent time off. After containing the patient, reassuring the other patients, and then speaking to the family, staff discovered that the patient had assaulted staff during several admissions, and

* *Clinical Nurse Specialist*
   Psychiatry Nursing Department, The Johns Hopkins Hospital

***Coordinator, Nursing Programs*
   Neuroscience and Psychiatry Departments, The Johns Hopkins Hospital

† *Director of Nursing*
   Neuroscience and Psychiatry Departments, The Johns Hopkins Hospital

†† *Clinical Outcomes Management Analyst*
   Department of Psychiatry, The Johns Hopkins Hospital

Clinical Nurse
   Psychiatry Nursing Department, The Johns Hopkins Hospital
   Clinical Instructor
   The Johns Hopkins University School of Nursing

Associate Professor, Psychiatry
   The Johns Hopkins University School of Medicine

always seemingly unprovoked. The staff expressed surprise and horror; this patient was known to have inflicted self-harm, but there was no knowledge of previous assault to others. Had the staff been made aware of his history, clear interventions would have been enacted medically as well as in nursing, including tapering the initial psychotropic when changing medications rather than discontinuing it, having PRNs available, more closely monitoring mood changes, and decreasing stimulation.

A team of nurses determined that the above scenario was a common occurrence, and decided to develop a plan of action. If staff, at the point of the patient admission, had more information about the patient's violence history and potential, a plan to reduce aggression could be immediately implemented. In addition, if a patient did exhibit aggressive behavior on the unit, detailed information—including the early plan of care, events precipitating aggression, and the type of aggression—could be trended to provide learning opportunities. These nurses created the tools that staff use today to learn more about patient aggression potential early in the hospitalization and provide plans to create a safer environment for patients and staff.

Background

Identification and skilled management of patients with aggression and agitation are growing safety concerns for psychiatric facilities as well as medical-surgical settings. Literature on psychiatric patient aggression emphasizes the importance of early assessment and identification of patient characteristics that may be indicative of aggression. Medical-surgical settings are beginning to document efforts that mirror those of psychiatric facilities in identifying and managing patient aggression. This chapter details a performance improvement initiative to enable nurses to identify patients who have a greater propensity for aggression and to implement appropriate interventions. The process involved a four-step approach using the Plan-Do-Study-Act model of performance improvement to investigate patient aggression through the development of aggression screening and incident tools. These instruments are intended to guide the treatment team to later evaluate the patient and revise planned interventions should an event occur during hospitalization.

Results

From October 2001 through mid-February 2003, approximately 41% of patients screened positive for an aggression history (first five elements of the aggression screen tool, Figure 10.1). There were 554 patient aggressive events. Ninety-two patients were involved in multiple aggressive events: 57 of those had two or three

Figure 10.1 Aggression Screening/Assessment Tool

THE JOHNS HOPKINS HOSPITAL
Department of Psychiatry

Aggression Screening/
Assessment Tool

Unit:_____

Date:

Legal History/Type of offense:

Date of last offense: _____

❑ **Unable to complete #1-12 due to patient acuity/condition. Complete within 48 hrs.**

❑ Assault/battery   ❑ Property damage
❑ Drug possession   ❑ Minor offense
❑ Other:_____

Do you own or have access to a gun?	Yes	No

Aggression History: (Circle Yes or No. Elaborate on all Yes responses)

1. Within the last five years have you

slapped/punched/kicked or hurt anyone?	Yes	No
threatened anyone with a weapon?	Yes	No
2. Have you ever hit or injured your parents/teacher/animals?	Yes	No
3. Have you ever hit anyone while a patient in the hospital?	Yes	No
4. Does being high/drunk play a role in your violent behavior?	Yes	No
5. Have you recently threatened anyone?	Yes	No

6. When was the last time any of the above occurred?_____

7. Do you hear voices now?	Yes	No
Do they tell you what to do?	Yes	No
8. Do you think others are trying to harm you?	Yes	No
9. Do you think others are trying to control you?	Yes	No
10. Is anyone or anything here on the unit bothering or irritating you now?	Yes	No
11. Are you having any thoughts to harm others?	Yes	No

12. How will we know you are angry and what do you do?_____

_____

What calms you when you are angry?_____

_____

Does the patient have a history of substance abuse?	Yes	No
Does the patient have a history of Cluster B?	Yes	No
Does the patient have a history of CO or Seclusion?	Yes	No (*Details*)_____

Patient's behavior during this interview (Circle all that apply):

sedated   confused   cooperative   irritable   guarded   uncooperative   resistant

Interviewer Signature and Title

If patient answered "yes" to any questions, check the appropriate planned interventions:

❑ Standing medications ordered for psychiatric symptoms
❑ PRN medications ordered for psychiatric symptoms
❑ Cognitive coping skills: thoughts vs. feelings
❑ Supportive therapy: decrease patient's subjective discomfort
❑ Anger management - addressed in daily session
❑ Limit setting - clear explanations of unit norms with reinforcements
❑ Planned staff presence in milieu: staff assigned to specific times
❑ Behavior Plan/Contact - written in the chart

❑ Q 15 minute checks
❑ Zoning
❑ Decreased patient stimulation-room restriction
❑ Constant Observation
❑ One to One
❑ Intensive Psychiatric Observation
❑ Admitted to Seclusion Room from ED
❑ Other:_____

events, 15 had four or five events, 12 had six to eight events, and 8 patients were involved in nine or more aggressive events. This is important information as we trend the elements of aggression that are common in patients with multiple aggressive events. The data indicate that appropriate care plans were implemented at time of admission for patients screened positive for violence history. Although events of aggression did not decrease over the reporting interval, events of injury to patients and staff were minimal and decreased over time.

Knowledge of a patient's aggression history is critical to the patient's effective treatment as well as prevention of untoward events. Information obtained from the screening instrument and from the aggression incident form has provided valuable data that influence treatment plans and help the nurse to anticipate aggressive behaviors, which will result in improved patient (and nurse) safety.

Plan

A challenging dimension of treating acutely ill psychiatric patients is the management of patient aggression by healthcare professionals during the course of inpatient hospitalizations. Since the early 1970s, researchers have engaged in efforts to understand precipitants of patient violence. Studies of psychiatric patient aggression address several key points: the impact of violence on the treatment setting; efforts to define patient variables that predict violent behavior; development of assessment instruments to screen for aggression predictors; and theoretical modeling to explain patient aggression. Through ongoing attempts to predict violent behavior, care providers can anticipate acts of aggression so that treatment efforts can be efficiently targeted at improving the mental health and functional life of seriously ill psychiatric patients. The consequences of patient aggression are not limited to psychiatric patients; they impact the work life and welfare of treatment teams in all acute care settings.

Clinicians have recognized that the antecedents of short-term violent behavior in hospitalized patients are not well understood. Exploration of this issue in recent decades has centered on direct assessment of psychiatric patient violence, through researcher-conducted interviews and record reviews.

Monahan (1982) poses critical questions and data that should be obtained in evaluating potential for violence:

- Precipitant events raising the question of violence potential and the context within which the events occurred
- Relevant demographic characteristics
- History of violent behavior
- Sources of stress in an individual's current environment and his or her ability to manage them violently or nonviolently
- Similarity between past contexts in which the person has coped violently and future contexts in which he or she will function

Monahan's thinking has prompted a gradual shift away from solely intuitive clinical judgments of dangerousness, toward statistical methods of prediction, as evidenced by studies published in the past 15 years (Monahan, 1982).

Owen et al. (1998) studied violent incidents in inpatient psychiatric settings among a group of repeatedly violent patients to understand the clinical and occupational health significance of repeated violence. They found that of the 175 patients involved in violent episodes, 12% were violence recidivists (the behavior reoccurs). These recidivists accounted for 69% of the 752 violent incidents identified. Tardiff et al. (1997) interviewed 763 patients admitted to a private psychiatric hospital to address three aims: to determine the rates of violence toward persons by patients before admission; to determine which types of patients are at greater risk of inflicting violence on other persons; and to describe the nature of the violent episodes in terms of target, location, weapon, and severity of injury. The study found that 14% of admitted patients had been violent toward other persons in the month before admission.

Harris and Rice (1997) reviewed selected studies on the prediction, management, and treatment of violent persons published in the last decade. They concluded that violence is predictable in some populations. The factors most highly and consistently related to risk are historical, including age, gender, past antisocial and violent conduct, psychopathy, aggressive childhood behavior, and substance abuse. They also state that actuarial methods are more accurate in predicting risk than unaided clinical judgment, which is a poor index.

The literature on patient aggression chronicles some efforts to use screening instruments to monitor aggressive behavior over time or to predict probability of violence. Yudofsky et al. (1986) use the Overt Aggression Scale (OAS) to measure aggressive behaviors in adults and children. The tool permits behaviors to be categorized into four levels, allows for the recording of specific interventions related to each aggressive event, and facilitates assessing events longitudinally for a single patient. The instrument's ratings are sensitive to changes in aggression that result from pharmacologic or other interventions, but the tool is not aggression-predictive in nature.

Swett and Mills's (1997) study evaluated three instruments as measures predictive of assaults that occurred during psychiatric hospitalization. On admission, the Mini Mental State Examination (MMSE) was administered to 335 acutely ill psychiatric patients, and diagnostic and demographic data were recorded. Immediately after admission, nurses rated the patients using the Nurses' Observational Scale for Inpatient Evaluation (NOSIE). Psychologists also rated the patients using the Brief Psychiatric Rating Scale (BPRS). Patients who committed assaults during hospitalization, and those who did not, were compared and relationships between several variables and assaults were evaluated statistically. The investigators found that a high score on the irritability factor of the NOSIE and failure to complete the MMSE correctly predicted the occurrence or nonoccurrence of assault 81% of the time.

Swanson et al. (1997) found that as the intensity or number of delusions increased, so did the risk of violence. Swanson also identified a combination of substance abuse and personality disorders as indicators.

More recently, the MacArthur Violence Risk Assessment Study followed over 1,000 recently discharged psychiatric patients for one year with a discharge interview and interviews every 10 weeks (Appelbaum, Robbins, & Monahan, 2000). Information was also obtained by collateral informants and official records. The researchers found that past violence and substance abuse were the two strongest predictors of violence in outpatients. They did not find that delusions were a predictor of violence in the outpatient population.

Johns Hopkins Hospital is a 900-bed tertiary academic hospital located in an urban, low socioeconomic area, with the associated problems of high unemployment, poor education, and a lack of general community resources, and with the psychosocial consequences of substance use. The psychiatric department has 88 beds located on 5 inpatient units with a large partial hospitalization population, composed of up to 50 general and specialty day hospital patients each day. Forty-five percent of the patient population admitted on three of the inpatient units self-report a history of aggression.

In response to nurses' concern that patients admitted to the hospital were becoming increasingly aggressive, one of the inpatient units developed a violence assessment tool. Nurses utilized the literature, their own experience with patients, and input from a staff forensic psychiatrist and the physician advisor. This tool assisted clinical nurses in identifying patients at risk for violence during their hospitalization and was completed on every patient admitted. Staff used the assessment tool to heighten their awareness of the patient's violence risk.

When the opportunity to revise the data collection tools associated with the use of restraints and seclusion surfaced, the goal was set to maximize the clinical usefulness of gathering data. The initial tool, which was utilized by one of the units, was revised to include a section that required the development of a plan to prevent aggression as well as updating the content based on a recent literature review. Prior to completing the planned interventions section of the tool, the assessment outcome was shared with the treatment team. The plan was developed with input from the team and individualized by identifying a variety of techniques from a defined menu. These strategies could include different levels of observation, coping strategies, and stress reduction. Emphasis was placed on the assessment/screen's importance in determining a patient's possible risk for aggressive behavior while in the hospital and ways to reduce that risk. Staff were instructed to use the assessment information to initiate a care plan designed to increase awareness of the patient's potential for escalation of aggressive behavior. Interventions were designed and implemented to prevent patient aggression by supporting the patient's own ability to remain in control.

Patient behaviors or characteristics have been examined in numerous studies in an attempt to determine if there are clear predictors of violence during a hospitalization, as referenced earlier in this article (Harris & Rice, 1997).

Command hallucinations and delusions that one is under threat and simultaneously being controlled by outside forces have been identified as other possible indicators. It was difficult to find clear cause-and-effect predictors of violence from a review of the literature, as the prevalence of violence is too low in the general population to infer specific characteristics. We wanted to find possible characteristics that would alert us of the need to have a plan to assist the patient to remain in control.

Do

The current assessment tool has undergone several revisions with changes based on literature findings and staff observations (Figure 10.1). Brevity and simplicity of completion are key considerations in creating a tool that will minimize the paperwork burden and ensure that every patient gets screened. Past legal history, history of violence, and antisocial traits are assessed, as well as the last time that the patient experienced legal difficulties or a violent outburst. Current delusions and hallucinations are ascertained, as is the content of these experiences. History of substance use, diagnosis of a personality disorder, and previous aggression while hospitalized are assessed by both patient questions and, if available, the patient's past medical history. Finally, the patient's level or ability to cooperate with the interview is noted. The admitting RN completes the Phipps Aggression Screening Tool (PAST, Figure 10.1) and initiates the plan section, developing an individualized treatment plan for that patient for any positive indicators. Further additions are made after the multidisciplinary treatment team meets. The original copy stays in the chart with a copy forwarded on for data collection.

By completing the tool for all aggressive occurrences we have identified that the majority of events do not require seclusion or restraint. This is important, as it begins to demonstrate the effectiveness of nursing interventions in the prevention of escalation, the utilization of the least restrictive interventions, and the prevention of violence. The Phipps Aggressive Patient Management Indicator (PAPMI, Figure 10.2) is completed by the RN when a patient has an aggressive or violent act, and becomes a permanent part of the chart, with a copy generated for data collection. Aggression is defined as forceful, goal-directed behavior that may be verbal or physical, and would include verbal threats towards objects or others, physical stances of anger, and the inability to follow safety requests. Violence is defined as outwardly directed destructive behavior.

The first section of the PAPMI is the plan of care, which duplicates the last question on the PAST. This helps to determine if the present plan is sufficient for the patient and identifies the least restrictive alternative interventions previously attempted. Treatment changes since admission are noted as well. Continuing with the tool, we want to identify precipitants to track any patterns that

Figure 10.2 Aggressive Patient Management Indicator

THE JOHNS HOPKINS HOSPITAL
Department of Psychiatric Nursing

Aggressive Patient Management Indicator
Peer Review/Confidential

For addressograph plate

Date_____ _____   Time_____   Unit_____

PREDETERMINED PLAN OF CARE (Check all that apply) delineated in chart or in treatment team rounds:

❑ Standing medications ordered for psychiatric symptoms
❑ PRN medications ordered for psychiatric symptoms
❑ Cognitive coping skills - thoughts vs feelings
❑ Supportive therapy - decrease patient's subjective discomfort
❑ Anger management - addressed in daily session
❑ Limit setting - clear explanations of unit norms with reinforcements
❑ Planned staff presence in milieu - staff assigned to specific times

❑ Behavior Plan/Contract - written in the chart
❑ Q 15 minute checks
❑ Zoning
❑ Decreased patient stimulation - room restriction
❑ Constant Observation
❑ One to One
❑ Intensive Psychiatric Observation
❑ Admitted to Seclusion Room from ED
❑ Other:_____

PRECIPITANT (Check all that apply)

❑ Food issues - quantity, menu
❑ Smoking issues
❑ Visitor/Family issues
❑ Peer issues
❑ Disagreement with treatment team expectations -
    staying out of room, attending groups
❑ Limits set
❑ Nondirectable behavior
❑ Psychotic symptoms - Hallucinations, delusions
❑ Cognitive impairment - Dementia, MR, formal thought disorder
❑ Other:_____

EVENT (Check all that apply)

❑ Verbal aggression/threats against other patients
❑ Verbal aggression/threats against staff
❑ Physical aggression against objects
❑ Physical aggression against self - non-lethal
❑ Physical aggression against self - lethal
❑ Physical aggression against staff
❑ Physical aggression against others
❑ Other_____
Briefly describe precipitant and event including
    medications given prior to event:_____
_____
_____

IMMEDIATE INTERVENTIONS POST-EVENT (Check all that apply)

❑ Verbal de-escalation techniques
❑ Verbal limit setting
❑ Planned staff presence in milieu
❑ Behavior plan/contract
❑ Patient placed on observation - Q 15 min. checks
❑ Patient placed on observation - zoning, CO
❑ Decrease patient stimulation/room restrict

❑ PRN medication given -_____
❑ Security active involvement
❑ Emergency bell activated
❑ Patient placed in Seclusion
❑ Patient placed on observation - 1:1, IPO
❑ Patient placed in restraints - 6-point vest, 4 point limb
❑ Other:_____

IMMEDIATE OUTCOME (Check all that apply)

❑ No longer verbally threatening
❑ Following staff directions
❑ Returns to normal tone of voice
❑ Nonverbal cues of violence ceased
❑ Processed with staff

❑ No change in behavior
❑ Escalation of behavior
❑ Improved but still threatening
❑ Discharged

STAFF SIGNATURE/TITLE

FORM # JHH-02-835-0002 (6/01)
Original - Place in patient's medical record;
Copies - RN completing original form will complete "Process Section". NCIII to complete Treatment Plan Revisions and forward Yellow
copy to the Nursing Office. Place Pink copy in Seclusion Log Book.

Figure 10.2   Continued

PROCESS (Check all Occurrences)

❏ A leader was identified
❏ The team processed the incident
❏ Individual nurse intervention
❏ The staff worked together as a team

❏ Emergency bell response was adequate   ❏ N/A
❏ Patient injury
❏ Staff injury

TREATMENT PLAN REVISIONS (check all that apply) Completed by NCIII in rounds - give copy to APM representative

❏ Behavior plan/contract
❏ Standing medication ordered for psychiatric symptoms
❏ Other:_____

❏ PRN medications ordered for psychiatric symptoms
❏ No change made

© The Johns Hopkins Hospital

we can alter, to further decrease the potential for violence. The event is then described as well as categorized. Immediate interventions and immediate outcome, which is defined as the outcome occurring within the next hour, are also identified. Other questions address our ability to appropriately and effectively deal with the aggressive incident following established aggressive patient management guidelines. Finally, the multidisciplinary treatment team discusses the aggressive or violent incident and changes, if appropriate, are made in the patient's treatment plan to decrease future incidents of aggression or violence.

Descriptors under each heading (Predetermined Plan, Precipitant, Event, Immediate Interventions, Immediate Outcome) are clustered by intensity of intervention or action. The rating of the behaviors is not part of the form, so that the RN completing it is not swayed by a predetermined classification. Nurse experts and a physician in the department completed the intensity clustering. An initial survey was sent out, and a subsequent meeting was held to discuss the rating criteria. The plan and interventions were clustered in severity as to actions the patient can demonstrate and the degree of control or assistance the staff needs to exert, from verbal interventions to observation to restraint use. The event was clustered around the division between verbal and physical aggression against others or objects. One of the key points stressed was the discussion of each aggressive event with the treatment team. This ensures that all aggressive events, major and minor, are profiled and that subsequent treatment plan revisions are based on a full picture of the patient's behaviors.

Study

The PAST was completed on 1,240 patient admissions from October 2001 to mid-February 2003. Of the 1,240 patients screened, the PAPMI was completed for 554 events caused by 92 patients.

Figure 10.3 Department of Psychiatry Admission Care Plan

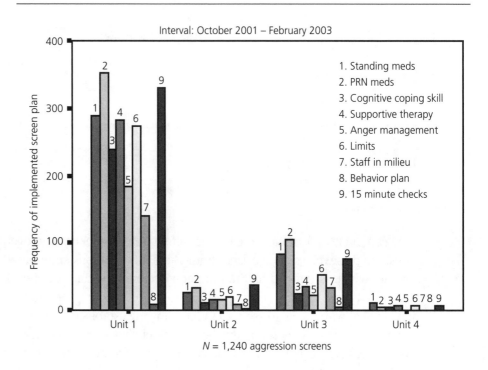

Interval: October 2001 – February 2003

1. Standing meds
2. PRN meds
3. Cognitive coping skill
4. Supportive therapy
5. Anger management
6. Limits
7. Staff in milieu
8. Behavior plan
9. 15 minute checks

N = 1,240 aggression screens

Figure 10.3 identifies the care plan interventions implemented at the time of admission. The data indicate that appropriate and least restrictive interventions are planned at admission for the unit-specific patient populations. More restrictive interventions, including more intense patient observations, are rarely implemented at admission. Figure 10.4 demonstrates the aggressive events per shift, with the largest number occurring on the day shift.

Figure 10.5a and 10.5b represent the frequency of interventions implemented after the aggressive event. The last four variable bars (emergency bell,

Figure 10.4 Department of Psychiatry Aggressive Events/Shift

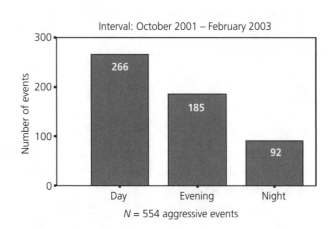

Interval: October 2001 – February 2003

N = 554 aggressive events

Figure 10.5a   Department of Psychiatry Interventions Implemented Post-event

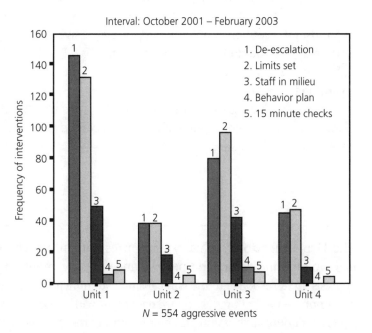

Figure 10.5b   Department of Psychiatry Interventions Implemented Post-event

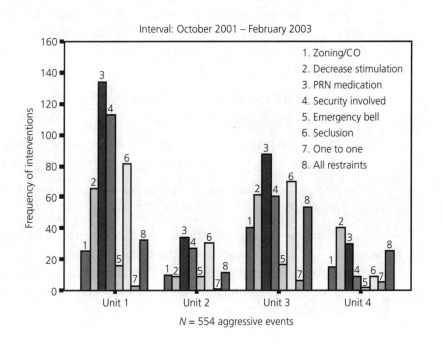

patient seclusion, one-to-one observation, and restraints) represent critical interventions. These variable-specific data are not mutually exclusive. Hence, multiple interventions may be implemented for each patient event. The data reflect that most interventions implemented for aggressive patient episodes were less restrictive. This demonstrates a positive finding related to our focus on patient rights and safety, which is consistent with earlier data observed by Dr. G. Jayaram et al. (2002).

As the database grows it will be helpful to note unit trends for the purpose of focused review to determine if the trends can be altered or if additional systems review is necessary.

Act

The Department of Psychiatry recognizes patient aggression as a high-risk, high-volume indicator. The performance improvement data collection and analysis are a response to the clinical staff's identification of the need to monitor and improve patient aggression management with a focus on safety outcomes.

The patient aggression screening and aggression event data are reported by nursing throughout the department. These data are summarized and reviewed quarterly by the Department of Psychiatry Aggressive Patient Management Committee, the Nursing Clinical Performance Improvement Committee, and the physician and nursing leadership.

Since the implementation of the aggression patient management tools, staff awareness of the potential for patient violence and the importance of early interventions has increased; however, reporting patient aggression can be a subjective experience for staff. The reporting threshold of the individual staff member varies greatly. Staff are encouraged to report all acts of patient aggression so we can develop an understanding of violence prevention methods and monitoring.

On a unit level, the data collection now serves as a treatment team communication tool to:

- identify patients at risk for violence
- plan interventions on admission
- review the precipitating factors associated with aggressive events
- evaluate and modify the interventions during the hospitalization
- review trends associated with aggressive events (i.e., shifts, patient populations)

The data also provide information for the department to justify and plan personnel and environmental resources, and have become a part of budget planning. Trends are monitored by the Aggressive Patient Management Committee to structure departmental education and identify needs for training support and revisions.

Conclusion

Healthcare providers across institutional settings are learning the importance of identifying patient aggression risk factors. This is no longer an issue that is confined to psychiatric settings. Nurses in general hospital settings are being injured by patient aggression in increasing numbers. Nielsen (1994) identified the need for medical-surgical nurses to perform early patient assessments upon admission by using a checklist of behavioral indicators. This activity triggered proactive patient care interventions and interdisciplinary team communication that resulted in decreased patient aggression and increased staff satisfaction.

The U.S. Department of Labor Occupational Safety and Health Administration (1998) published work practice guidelines to assist in aggression prevention. These guidelines apply to all patient care settings and include opportunities for aggression assessment and intervention at the beginning of the patient hospitalization:

- Inform the patient and family/significant others that aggression is not tolerated.

- Assess the patient's behavioral history related to aggression toward others.

- Provide and ensure that staff participate in aggressive patient management training.

Early identification of patients at risk using an aggression assessment tool is an important step toward planning appropriate prevention measures. This is also an opportunity for patients and family to be informed of the hospital's philosophy and response to patient aggression.

There are many research questions yet to be answered. The PAST and the PAPMI are works in progress. The data generate ongoing interdisciplinary discussions about the most efficient ways to train staff, intervene early, and prevent patient aggression. Inter-rater reliability needs to be established for the PAST.

Clearly, the most important opportunity to reduce patient aggression rests with the bedside clinicians. In addition to all of their patient responsibilities, including assessment, management of aggression, and documentation, they are being asked to increase their documentation to provide crucial patient aggression data. Staff must be informed about data analysis results and departmental improvement strategies to reinforce efforts to ensure a safe environment.

References

Appelbaum, P., Robbins, P. C., & Monahan, J. (2000). Violence and delusions: Data from the MacArthur violence risk assessment study. *American Journal of Psychiatry, 157*(4), 566–572.

Harris, G. T., & Rice, M. E. (1997). Risk appraisal and management of violent behavior. *Psychiatric Services, 48*(9), 1168–1176.

Jayaram, G., Dunn, G., Taylor, K., Brannan, D., & Keenan, B. (2002). Aggression screening to predict and prevent use of seclusion in acutely ill patients. Abstract. American Psychiatric Association.

Monahan, J. (1982). Clinical prediction of violent behavior. *Psychiatric Annals, 12*(5), 509–513.

Nielsen, J. (1994). Preventing violence in the hospital: A nursing unit's quality improvement story. *QRC Advisor, 11*(1) 1–8.

Owen, C., Tarantello, C., Jones, M., & Tennant, C. (1998). Repetitively violent patients in psychiatric units. *Psychiatric Services, 49*(11), 1458–1461.

Swanson, J., Estroff, S., Swartz, M., Borum, R., Lachicotte, W., Zimmer, C., & Wagner, R. (1997). Violence and severe mental disorder in clinical and community populations: The effects of psychotic symptoms, comorbidity, and lack of treatment. *Psychiatry, 60*(1), 1–22.

Swett, C., & Mills, T. (1997). Use of the NOSIE to predict assaults among acute psychiatric patients. *Psychiatric Services, 48*(9), 1177–1180.

Tardiff, K., Marzuk, P. M., Leon, A. C., Portera, L., & Weiner, C. (1997). Violence by patients admitted to a private psychiatric hospital. *American Journal of Psychiatry, 154*(1), 88–93.

U.S. Department of Labor Occupational Safety and Health Administration. (1998). Guidelines for Preventing Workplace Violence for Health Care and Social Service Workers.

Yudofsky, S. C., Silver, J. M., Jackson, W., Endicott, J., & Williams, D. (1986). The overt scale for the objective rating of verbal and physical aggression. *American Journal of Psychiatry, 143*(1), 35–39.

CHAPTER 11

Resources for Conducting a Safety Project

Sharon Strobel, RN, M.S.

You have been a staff nurse on a 42-bed pediatric medical-surgical unit for 4 years. A significant component of the patient population includes children suffering from reactive airway disease exacerbations and asthma. You have noticed that whenever children respond poorly to frequent nebulization therapy, the physicians order transfer to the pediatric intensive care unit (PICU) for intravenous magnesium administration. You know from past experience that transfers have been delayed while the shift coordinator worked to make a bed available. This delayed maximizing bronchodilation therapy, which could have had a negative effect on the patient clinically, increased hospital costs, stressed the patient and family, and potentially increased the patient's length of stay. In discussions with your peers, you have heard "this is the way it is always done." Because your nursing unit has 5 designated intermediate care beds (IMC) where the nurse–patient ratio is lower than for the remaining 37 beds, you have begun to question the rationale for using the PICU rather than IMC beds for intravenous magnesium therapy for bronchodilation. You wonder whether there are identifiable safety issues and if any resources are available to help review the policies and procedures associated with the clinical care of this patient population.

Many processes we use in health care have become routine, accepted, and performed without questioning the evidence surrounding them. The good news is that when these questions arise, a variety of internal and external resources can now be quickly accessed to answer the questions as they emerge. It is a matter of knowing what these resources are and how to access them.

Internal sources may include policies and procedures (and their references); experts on the patient population, safety, and risk management; the library; and the organization's intranet. You could also review internal communications from the facility's administrators, as well as medical and nursing leadership groups, to determine the pressing issues. Discussions with peers, leaders, or managers may help to focus your actions. Review of safety projects already conducted within your organization may provide additional guidance in developing and carrying out your ideas. Confer with nurse researchers or faculty with research experience to further define your activities.

In addition to the organization's internal resources, extensive external sources are available that can provide a rich source of trends, evidence-based clinical practice, and benchmarking data. Review guidelines, publications, and safety data from local, state, and federal government agencies. Explore the private sector for performance and safety measures as well as quality indicators. Investigate professional medical and nursing organizations and associations for evidence-based clinical practice recommendations. Utilize the library to review the literature. Probe the Internet with broad queries; explore links and narrow your search as you traverse the World Wide Web.

Safety resources have become more prevalent and accessible for nurses. In the example presented, potential resources would include literature searches on asthma management for the pediatric population, including the use of magnesium. Potential sources of information that the team should consider include CINAHL, MedWeb, Medline, the TRIP Database, and the Cochrane Center and Collaboration web site. Focused review should also include the Centers for Disease Control and Prevention, the National Institutes of Health (NIH) Health Information Index, the Food and Drug Administration Med Watch, the National Guideline Clearinghouse, the National Library of Medicine, and the Institute for Safe Medication Practices (ISMP). Start with a broad concept or question and narrow the search as you gather evidence to support special clinical practice. The team may also consider contacting other medical facilities to ask about their standards for clinical practice.

The availability of high quality safety resources will foster the progress of a safety project. Knowing how to access these resources will arm nurses with a compendium of knowledge and expert contacts that they can use in their own work.

The objective of this chapter is to help nurse leaders identify safety-related internal and external resources that can provide information and guidance when conducting a safety project. The resources that follow are divided into government resources, drug information, medical and nursing directories, indexes, clinical resources, professional organizations and associations, research, miscellaneous safety sites, and Search Engines, and include the web site address.

City, State, and Federal Government Resources

- Baltimore City Health Department: http://www.baltimorecity.gov

- Centers for Disease Control and Prevention (CDC): http://www.cdc.gov

- Centers for Disease Control National Nosocomial Infections Surveillance (CDC NNIS)—epidemiology information, nosocomial rates, and resistance trends useful for benchmarking: http://www.cdc.gov/ncidod/hip/health_reports.htm

- Center for Medicare and Medicaid Services (CMS)—[formerly Health Care Financing Administration (HCFA)]—provides a monthly newsletter in HTML and PDF formats; includes resources on broad patient safety issues under the *Medicare* and *Professional and technical publications* headings, as well as quality of care information that provides interpretation of new standards designed to improve patient safety and compliance: http://www.hcfa.gov

- Florida Hospital Association (FHA)—resources include products and services, reports and publications, with additional links to state, federal, managed care, children's, workforce and news resources: http://www.fha.org

- Food and Drug Administration Med Watch—includes med error reports, specific drugs related to errors, and federal guidelines: http://www.fda.gov

- Maryland Board of Nursing: http://www.mbon.org

- Maryland Department of Health & Mental Hygiene: http://www.dhmh.state.md.us

- NASA Human Factors Research and Technology Division—links to library resources utilizing "human factors" advanced search: http://www.nasa.gov

- National Cancer Institute: http://www.cancer.gov

- National Center for Patient Safety (NCPS) (located under the Department of Veterans Affairs)—patient safety self-learning lessons on Healthcare Failure Mode and Effects Analysis (HFMEA), "Root Cause Analysis (RCA)" and "Triage": http://www.patientsafety.gov

- National Guideline Clearinghouse—comprehensive database of evidence-based clinical practice guidelines, related documents, and links produced by the Agency for Healthcare Research and Quality (AHRQ) in partnership with the American Medical Association (AMA) and American Association of Health Plans (AAHP): http://www.guideline.gov

- National Information Center on Health Services Research and Health Care Technology (NICHSR): http://www.nlm.nih.gov/nichsr

- National Institutes of Health (NIH) Health Information Index: http://www.nih.gov. See also: http://health.nih.gov

- National Library of Medicine, NLM Gateway—web-based system allowing simultaneous search of multiple databases at the National Library of Medicine (NLM): http://www.ncbi.nlm.nih.gov/pubmed

- Office of Inspector General (OIG)—updates on compliance issues and CMS/HCFA; JCAHO report regarding survey changes: http://www.os.dhhs.gov/oig

- U.S. Department of Health and Human Services (DHHS): http://www.os.dhhs.gov

- VA Healthcare Network, Upstate New York, includes VISN2 Network Policy—integrated patient safety/risk management program components (incident reporting, flow charts for reportable events, and root cause analysis for specific sentinel events): http://www.va.gov/VISNS/visn02/network_nf.html

- Virtual Learning Center and Patient Safety—dozens of self-learning modules involving patient safety (nonpunitive patient safety, wrong-site surgery, restraints), a slide show and information downloads: http://www.va.gov/med/osp/cgi-bin/patientsafety_intronew_int.asp

- World Health Organization (WHO): http://www.who.int

Drug Information

- *MEDLINEplus Drug Information*—from National Library of Medicine: http://medlineplus.gov

- *Medscape DrugInfo:* http://www.medscape.com

- *MICROMEDEX*—comprehensive drug database: http://www.micromedex.com

- *RxList*—top 200 prescribed drugs, search by imprint codes: http://www.rxlist.com

- U.S. Phamacopoeia (USP)—major drug standards-setting organization, medication monographs: http://www.usp.org

Medical and Nursing Directories, Indexes, and Clinical Resources

- All Nurses—a compilation of numerous nursing web sites with links: http://www.allnurses.com

- American Nurse: http://www.nursingworld.org

- ANNA*Link*—official web site of the American Nephrology Nurses's Association (ANNA): http://anna.inurse.com

- CancerNet: http://www.cancer.gov
- Cancer Nursing—a comprehensive source about oncology disease, treatment, news, research, clinical trial information, message boards, and support groups: http://www.CancerSourceRN.com
- CINAHL—a nursing and allied health database of information and resources for healthcare professionals: http://www.cinahl.com
- Doctor's Guide: http://www.docguide.com
- Emergency Nursing World—a comprehensive practice-based resource of full text articles, research, Internet resource links, and discussion groups: http://enw.org
- Emory University's Med Web—a catalog of biomedical and health-related web sites maintained by the Robert W. Woodruff Health Sciences Center Library: http://whsc.emory.edu
- Evidence Based Health Care Project, University of Minnesota: http://evidence.ahc.umn.edu/ebn.htm
- Evidence-Based Nursing: http://www.ebn.bmjjournals.com
- Galaxy Medicine: http://www.MedWebPlus.com/obj/4285
- Hardin Meta Directory, Nursing: http://www.lib.uiowa.edu/hardin/md/
- Healthfinder: http://www.healthfinder.gov
- HealthGate Information Systems: http://www.healthgate.com
- HealthLinks—an online health care information portal which includes a directory and guide to health information: http://www.healthlinks.net
- HealthWeb—an interface providing organized access to evaluated, non-commercial, Internet-accessible resources: http://www.healthweb.org
- Johns Hopkins University School of Nursing: http://www.son.jhmi.edu
- *Journal of Issues in Nursing*: http://www.nursingworld.org/ojin
- Martindale's Health Science Guide: http://www.martindalecenter.com/HSG/HSGuide.html
- Martindale's Virtual Nursing Center—an extensive collection of nursing web sites with links: http://www.martindalecenter.com
- MDConsult—reference books, journals, practice guidelines, patient education handbooks, drug information, and industry news. Personal edition requires membership: http://www.mdconsult.com. Generic edition does not require membership: http://www.library.ucsf.edu/db/mdconsult.html
- *MEDLINE* available through Medscape by WebMD—clinical and nursing index of articles: http://www.medscape.com
- Medical Matrix—a directory of selected clinical resources with a primary audience of healthcare professionals; requires registration: http://www.medmatrix.org
- Miscellaneous nursing links: http://www.Cybernurse.com

- National Center for Emergency Medicine Informatics: http://www.ncemi.org
- National Council of State Boards of Nursing: http://www.ncsbn.org
- National Guideline Clearinghouse: http://www.guideline.gov
- Nightingale, University of Tennessee College of Nursing, Knoxville—an extensive compilation of nursing resources with web site links: http://w3.one.net/~gloriamc/nurse.html
- Nurse Healer—complementary and alternative nursing: http://www.nursehealer.com
- Nurse Linx—a news service that scans medical and nursing news daily to locate top articles and reports, categorizing them into subspecialties: http:www.NurseLinx.com
- NurseNet—an open, global electronic conference site for discourse about diverse nursing issues, including administration, education, practice and research nursing: http://www.graduateresearch.com/NurseNet
- Nurse Practitioner Central—resources and web site links for nurse practitioners: http://www.npcentral.net
- NurseWeek—a general information web site with Internet links for nurses: http://www.nurseweek.com
- Nursing association web search guide: http://www.Allnurses.com/Associations
- Nursing Center—links to journals, clinical guidelines, online education; requires membership: http://www.nursingcenter.com
- Nursing Internet Resources, Adelaide University—information about and instructions for accessing internet resources: http://www.library.adelaide.edu.au/guide/med/nursing/
- Nursing World, American Nurses' Association (ANA)—lists ANA publications, full text articles, continuing education, legislative information, fact sheets, and position papers; excellent links to nursing Internet sites: http://www.ana.org
- Nursing, Midwifery and Allied Health Professionals (NMAP)—a UK-based searchable gateway to evaluated, quality Internet sources, aimed at students, researchers, health and medical practitioners and academics: http://www.nmap.ac.uk
- Oregon Evidence-Based Practice Center—source of systematic reviews of healthcare topics: http://www.ohsu.edu/epc
- Oregon Health Sciences University, Patient Education Resources, English and non-English sites: http://www.ohsu.edu/library/consumerhealth
- Publishers for the National Academies: http://books.nap.edu

- School of Health Science, University of Birmingham—(formerly NURSE), a UK-based searchable nursing information service: http://medweb.bham.ac.uk/nursing

- Slack, Inc. Nursing Internet Resources (Health Information Management and Education Company): http://www.slackinc.com/areas.asp

- Springhouse Reference Library: http://www.nursingcenter.com

- The Institute for Johns Hopkins Nursing: http://www.ijhn.jhmi.edu

- The Joanna Briggs Institute—libraries and resources for evidence-based nursing practice: http://www.joannabriggs.edu.au/about/home.php

- *The Lancet*: http://www.thelancet.com/journal

- The Virtual Hospital, University of Iowa—information for healthcare professionals: http://www.vh.org

- The WWW Virtual Library—Medicine and Health: http://londonbridge.ohsu.edu/wwwvl/

- University of Texas Medical Branch (UTMB)—links to patient safety organizations and information: http://www.utmb.edu/patientsafety

- Virtual Nursing College, Langara College, British Columbia: http://www.langara.bc.ca/vnc

- Welch Medical Library, Johns Hopkins University—Consumer Health and Patient Information Resources: http://www.welch.jhu.edu/internet/quicklinks.html

- WholeNurse Alternative and Holistic WebCenters—a guide to alternative and holistic health care Internet resources: http://www.wholenurse.com

Professional Organizations and Associations

- Academy of Medical-Surgical Nurses (AMSN): http://www.medsurgnurse.org

- Accreditation Association for Ambulatory Health Care (AAAHC): http://www.aaahc.org

- Agency for Healthcare Research and Quality (AHRQ) (formerly AHCPR, Agency for Health Care and Policy and Research)—site of critical analysis of patient safety practices: http://www.ahrq.gov (agency site).
  See also: http://www.ahrq.gov/clinic/ptsafety/spotlight.htm and http://www.ahrq.gov/qual/errorsix.htm

- American Academy of Ambulatory Care Nursing (AAACN): http://www.aaacn.org

- American Academy of Nurse Practitioners: http://www.aanp.org
- American Academy of Nursing (AAN): http://www.nursingworld.org
- American Association of Ambulatory Surgery Centers (AAASC): http://www.aaasc.org
- American Association of Colleges of Nursing (AACN): http://www.aacn.nche.edu
- American Association of Critical Care Nurses (AACCN): http://www.aacn.org
- American Association for Neuroscience Nurses (AANN)—links to abstracts from *The Journal of Neuroscience Nursing*: http://www.aann.org
- American Association of Nurse Anesthetists (AANA)—focuses on anesthesia safety, patient communication, conscious sedation, and standards of safety: http://www.aana.com
  See also: http://www.anesthesiapatientsafety.com
- American Association of Occupational Health Nurses (AAOHN): http://www.aaohn.org
- American Association of PeriAnesthesia Nurses: http://www.aspan.org
- American Association of Poison Control Centers (AAPCC): http://www.aapcc.org
- American Association of Spinal Cord Injury Nurses: http://www.aascin.org
- American Cancer Society: http://www.cancer.org
- American College of Medical Quality (ACMQ): http://www.acmq.org
- American College of Nurse Midwives: http://www.midwife.org
- American College of Nurse Practitioners: http://www.nurse.org/acnp
- American Heart Association: http://www.americanheart.org
- American Holistic Nurses Association: http://www.ahna.org
- American Hospital Association (AHA)—site of medication error information and resources: http://www.aha.org
- American Hospital Association News—offers information on AHA initiatives and focuses on medication safety and safety culture; includes links to major reports and successful practices: http://www.ahanews.com
- American Medical Association (AMA)—site directs you to the National Patient Safety Foundation web site (http://www.npsf.org); you can pull up AMA-related reports and articles through search: http://www.ama-assn.org
- American National Standards Institute (ANSI) Healthcare Informatics Standards Board: http://web.ansi.org
- American Nephrology Nurses Association (ANNA): http://anna.org

- American Nurses Association (ANA)—focuses on workplace and OSHA issues: http://www.ana.org
- American Organization of Nurse Executives—general announcements and statements related to patient safety; information on patient safety fellowship: http://www.aone.org
- American Osteopathic Association (AOA): http://www.osteopathic.org
- American Psychiatric Nurses Association (APNA): http://www.apna.org
- American Public Health Association (APHA): http://www.apha.org
- American Radiologic Nurses Association: http://www.arna.net
- American Society for Healthcare Risk Management (ASHRM)—multiple resources, publications, summary, and tracking of federal and state legislation: http://www.ashrm.org
- American Society of Health-System Pharmacists (ASHP): http://www.ashp.com
  See also: http://www.ashp.com/patient_safety
- American Society of Law, Medicine & Ethics (ASLME): http://www.aslme.org
- American Society for Healthcare Risk Management: http://www.ashrm.org
- Anesthesia Patient Safety Foundation (APSF)—clinical information, newsletters, and safety links: http://www.apsf.org
- Armed Forces Institute of Pathology: http://www.afip.org
- Association for Hospital Medical Education (AHME): http://ahme.org
- Association of American Medical Colleges (AAMC): http://www.aamc.org
- Association of Nurses in AIDS Care: http://www.anacnet.org
- Association of Pediatric Oncology Nurses (APON): http://www.apon.org
- Association of PeriOperative Registered Nurses (AORN): http://www.aorn.org
- Association for Professionals in Infection Control and Epidemiology (APIC)—information on patient safety training, tools for effective strategies for improving patient safety, and resources: http://www.apic.org
- Association of Rehabilitation Nurses (ARN): http://www.rehabnurse.org
- Association of Women's Health, Obstetric & Neonatal Nurses (AWHONN): http://www.awhonn.org
- Blue Cross and Blue Shield Association (BCBSA): http://www.bluecares.com
- Case Management Society of America: http://www.cmsa.org

- Center for the Evaluative Clinical Sciences at Dartmouth Medical School—locus of scientists and clinicians focusing on evaluating practice of medicine: http://dartmouth.edu/~cecs/

- Dermatology Nurses Association: http://www.dna.inurse.com

- Emergency Care Research Institute (ECRI)—abstracts on medical device reports and recommendations; range of tools and resources related to safety and healthcare quality: http://www.ecri.org (agency) and Medical Device Safety Reports: http://www.mdsr.ecri.org

- Emergency Nurses Association (ENA): http://www.ena.org

- Endocrine Nurses Society: http://www.endo-nurses.org

- Home Healthcare Nurses Association: http://www.nahc.org/hhna

- Hospice & Palliative Nurses Association: http://www.hpna.org

- International Association of Forensic Nurses: http://www.forensicnurse.org

- Intravenous Nurses Society: http:www.ins1.org

- Institute for Healthcare Improvement—site of best practices, administrative, and breakthrough clinical innovations information, including downloadable resources; linked to National Coalition of Health Care; provides links to Hospital Infections Program, APIC, and CDC: http://www.ihi.org (agency).

- Institute of Medicine (IOM) (also known as National Academy of Sciences Institute of Medicine)—reports aimed at culture of safety of organization: http://www.iom.edu
  See also: http://www.national-academies.org

- Institute for Safe Medication Practices (ISMP)—independent organization focusing on medication error reporting and reduction; provides medication alerts, and communication tools for pharmacists: http://www.ismp.org

- Interagency Council on Information Resources for Nursing (ICIRN): http://www.icirn.org

- Joint Commission on Accreditation of Healthcare Organizations (JCAHO)—new patient safety standards; description of sentinel events, reporting database, root cause analysis, and current summary report of findings: http://www.jcaho.org

- Leukemia and Lymphoma Society: http://www.leukemia.org

- Massachusetts Coalition for the Prevention of Medical Errors (MCPME)—best practice recommendations for medication error reduction; patient medication guide: http://www.macoalition.org

- Massachusetts Hospital Association (MHA), Massachusetts Coalition for Prevention of Medical Errors—basic patient safety information and resources; summaries of foundations and functions; extensive list of publications, including best practice recommendations, medication errors, and tools for leadership: http://www.mhalink.org/mcpme/mcpme_welcome.htm

- National Association of Children's Hospitals and Related Institutions (NACHRI): http://www.nachri.org
- National Academies: http://www.nationalacademies.org See also: http://www.iom.edu
- National Association of Boards of Pharmacy (NABP): http://www.nabp.net
- National Association of Clinical Nurse Specialists (NACNS): http://www.nacns.org
- National Association for Healthcare Quality (NAHQ)—organization for healthcare quality professionals; links to *Journal for Healthcare Quality*: http://www.nahq.org
- National Association of Neonatal Nurses (NANN): http://www.nann.org
- National Association of Orthopedic Nurses (NAON): http://www.orthonurse.org
- National Association of Pediatric Nurse Associates & Practitioners, Inc.: http://www.napnap.org
- National Association of School Nurses: http://www.nasn.org
- National Black Nurses Association, Inc.: http://www.nbna.org
- National Coalition of Health Care (NCHC)—information, press releases, and speeches related to patient care/safety initiatives: http://www.nchc.org
- National Committee for Quality Assurance (NCQA): http://www.ncqa.org
- National Coordinating Council for Medication Error Reporting and Prevention (NCCMERP)—collaborative council of 10 national organizations aimed at identifying causes of medication errors and promoting safe medication use: http://www.nccmerp.org
- National Council of State Boards of Nursing, Inc. (NCSBN): http://www.ncsbn.org
- National Federation of Licensed Practical Nurses, Inc.: http://www.nflpn.org
- National Gerontologic Nursing Association (NGNA): http://www.ngna.org
- National League for Nursing (NLN): http://www.nln.org
- National Nurses Society on Addictions: http://www.nnsa.org
- National Nursing Staff Development Organization: http://www.nnsdo.org

- National Patient Safety Foundation (NPSF)—major site of patient safety sponsored by AMA; provides organizational links, and is a source of pertinent literature: http://www.npsf.org

- National Quality Forum(NQF)/National Forum on Healthcare Quality Measurement—organization initiating a measurement project focused on identifying and developing concensus on a core set of safety measurements related to avoidable, serious events in hospital care; goal of standardization of data collection and reporting of events within and across states: http://www.qualityforum.org

- North American Nursing Diagnosis Association (NANDA): http://www.nanda.org

- Oncology Nursing Society: http://www.ons.org

- Partnership for Patient Safety—promotes patient-centered approach for improving health care: http://www.p4ps.org

- Patient Safety Institute (PSI)—promotes the use of technology and the development of relationships to reduce medical errors in hospitals: http://www.ptsafety.org

- Pediatric Pharmacy Advocacy Group: http://www.ppag.org

- Quality Interagency Coordination Task Force (QuIC)—developed AHRQ report: *Doing What Counts for Patient Safety: Federal Actions to Reduce Medical Errors and Their Impact*; provides framework for types of errors; in downloadable form or online: http://www.quic.gov
  See also: http://www.usp.org

- Risk Management Foundation (RMF)—links to interview with safety guru Lucian Leape; online CME course on risk management; eight principles for developing education in patient safety and other resources: http://www.rmf.harvard.edu

- Sigma Theta Tau International Honor Society of Nursing: http://www.nursingsociety.org

- Society for Vascular Nursing: http://www.svnnet.org

- Society of Gastroenterology Nurses & Associates, Inc.: http://www.sgna.org

- Society of Pediatric Nurses (SPN): http://pedsnurses.org

- Society of Trauma Nurses (STN): http://www.nursingsociety.org

- Society of Urologic Nurses & Associates: http://www.suna.org

- The Hospital and Health System Association of Pennsylvania (HAP): http://www.haponline.org/quality/safety

- Transcultural Nursing Society: http://www.tcns.org

- Virginians Improving Patient Care and Safety (VIPCS)—extensive listing of organizations and links to specific fact sheets; patient's guide; "net tracker" link to new items: http://www.vipcs.org
- Wound, Ostomy & Continence Nurses Society: http://www.wocn.org

Research

- Center for Research Support (CeReS): http://www.ceres.uwcm.ac.uk/
- CenterWatch: Clinical Trials Listing Service: http://www.centerwatch.com
- Clinical Calculators and Medical E-Tools, Welch Medical Library, Johns Hopkins University: http://www.welch.jhu.edu/internet/quicklinks.html
- Clinical Trials—government sponsored: http://www.ClinicalTrials.gov
- Clinical Trials—miscellaneous: http://www.clinicaltrials.com
- Cochrane Center and Collaboration, Database of Systematic Reviews—searchable database of systematic reviews of clinical interventions and treatments: http://www.cochrane.org
- Community of Science Web Server: http://www.cos.com
- Computer Retrieval of Information on Scientific Projects (CRISP)—searchable database of federally funded biomedical research projects: https://www.crisp.cit.nih.gov
- Health Statistics—a guide to locating health statistics on the web: http://www.hsls.pitt.edu/intres/guides/statclow.html
- Illinois Researcher Information Service (IRIS)—search engine for funding opportunities through the IRIS system: http://www.library.uiuc.edu/iris/
- Johns Hopkins University Center for Nursing Research: http://www.son.jhmi.edu/research/CNR
- Johns Hopkins University School of Medicine Clinical Trials Unit: http://www.jhmi.edu
- Middlesex University, London, Teaching/Learning Resources for Evidence-Based Practice—web-site tutorials for teaching the five steps of evidence-based practice: www.mdx.ac.uk/www/rctsh/ebp/main.htm
- Midwest Nursing Research Society (MNRS): http://www.mnrs.org
- National Information Center on Health Services Research and Health Care Technology—large list of healthcare research sites

arranged alphabetically and by subject:
www.nlm.nih.gov/nichsr/nichsr.html

■ National Institute of Nursing Research (NINR), a branch of National Institutes of Health—NIH nursing research information:
http://www.nih.gov/ninr/links.html

■ Nightingale—links and information on research, practice, education, publications, and other resources:
http://w3.one.net/~gloriamc/nurse.html

■ Registry of Nursing Research, Sigma Theta Tau:
http://www.nursingsociety.org/research/main.html

■ Research instrument resources:
http://www.indstate.edu/nurs/mary/tool.htm

■ Statistics, Welch Medical Library, Johns Hopkins University:
http://www.welch.jhu.edu/reference/statistics.html

■ University of Rochester Medical Center—web-based tutorial focusing on the five steps of evidence-based practice:
http://www.urmc.rochester.edu/hslt/miner/resources/researchers/index.cfm

Miscellaneous Safety Sites

■ ABCs of Patient Safety: http://www.npsf.org/html/abcs.html

■ Agency for Health Care Policy and Research (AHCPR)—Medical Errors & Patient Safety Subdirectory Page; information about AHCPR's efforts to reduce medical errors and improve patient safety: http://www.ahcpr.gov/qual/errorsix.htm

■ American Academy of Family Physicians—healthcare quality assessment: http://www.aafp.org/index.html

■ Annenberg Center for Health Sciences: http://www.annenberg.net

■ AORN Patient Safety First—site devoted to patient safety:
http://www.patientsafetyfirst.org

■ Bad Human Factors Designs—human factors in design:
http://www.baddesigns.com

■ Bridge Medical, The Patient Safety Company—helps hospitals and health systems prevent medication administration, transfusion, and lab specimen collection errors; activities aimed at increasing effectiveness through clinical decision-making support at point of care; extensive listing of conferences, trade shows, events aimed at addressing patient safety, and developing solutions:
http://www.bridgemedical.com

- Center for Proper Medication Use—site offers practical information related to medication safety, including herbal and OTC; products include videos, brochures, and consumer guides: http://www.cpmu.org

- Children's Patient Safety Learning Center: http://www.childrensonline.org/safety

- CNN: http://www.cnn.com

- Comprehensive Health Enhancement Support System (CHESS)—mission is research, development, and dissemination of health communication technologies to optimize health behaviors, quality of life, and use of resources: http://chess.chsra.wisc.edu/Chess

- Current Research in Patient Safety—review of current research on patient safety underway in the United States: http://www.npsf.org/html/current_research.html

- Health Forum: http://www.healthforum.com

- Human Factors Research Project (formerly Aerospace Crew Research Project): http://www.homepage.psy.utexas.edu/homepage/group/HelmreichLAB/

- Institute for Safe Medication Practices (ISMP): http://www.ismp.org

- MedErrors, Bridge Medical Inc.—site devoted to providing information on medication errors and adverse drug reactions in hospitals; links to experts and resources: http://www.mederrors.com

- Medical Error Reduction and Patient Safety—extensive references, products, and services as well as links to sites aimed at reduction of medical errors and improvement of patient safety: http://www.medicalerrorreduction.com

- National Patient Safety Foundation (NPSF)—patient safety bibliography; links to review literature on patient safety: http://www.npsf.org/html/bibliography.html

- Patient Safety Reporting Systems—provides information on centers of patient inquiry and a medication error reporting system modeled after the NASA reporting program; program is in effect in VA facilities: http://psrs.arc.nasa.gov/program_background.htm

- Patient Safety Resources: http://www.informatics-review.com/safety.html

- Premier, Inc.—links to extensive patient safety resources including summaries of issues, guidelines, regulations, and forms; an annotated bibliography of resources and links; and sample tools: http://www.premierinc.com/frames/index.jsp?pagelocation=/all/safety/resources/

- Quality Indicator Project, The Association of Maryland Hospitals and Healthsystems (MHA): http://www.qiproject.org

- Robert L. Helmreich home page:
  http://www.psy.utexas.edu/psy/helmreich/nasaut.htm
- Sentara Patient Safety Center:
  http://www.sentara.com/explorehealth
- Vaccine Adverse Event Reporting System (VAERS)—post-marketing safety surveillance program collecting information on adverse events related to vaccine administration:
  http://www.fda.gov/cber/vaers/vaers.htm
- VHA, Inc.: http://www.vha.com
- Yale New Haven Health Safety Center:
  http://www.yalenewhavenhealth.org/healthtopics/safety.htm

Search Engines

- AltaVista: http://www.altavista.com
- Ask Jeeves: http:www.askjeeves.com
- Excite: http:www.excite.com
- Google: Health/Nursing Directory of web sites: http://directory.google.com/Top/Health/Nursing
- HealthWeb: http://www.healthweb.org
- InfoSeek: http://www.infoseek.com
- LookSmart: http://www.looksmart.com
- Lycos: http://www.lycos.com
- Medscape by WebMD: http://www.medscape.com
- MedHunt: http://www.hon.ch/MedHunt/
- MSN Search Service: http://search.msn.com
- Northern Light—good site for researchers; large index of items with special collections not available from other search engines:
  www.nlsearch.com
- The TRIP Database—searches multiple sites with hyperlinks to evidence-based material on the web: http://www.miart.co.uk/I-medicine.info/search_Trip_database.htm
- Yahoo, Health/Nursing Directory: http://www.yahoo.com

The Johns Hopkins Hospital Performance Improvement Workbook

The Johns Hopkins Hospital Performance Improvement Workbook

At the Johns Hopkins Hospital (JHH), we are always trying to improve our processes to achieve better outcomes. Teamwork is the key to our success. This workbook is designed to assist teams in identifying, developing, and implementing performance improvement (PI) projects. First, we have included a worksheet to guide you through the process. Next, we have provided more detail in the appendices.

Model for Improvement: PDSA

What are we trying to accomplish?

Who should be on the team to make this happen? (Team leaders, members, staff support)
•
•
•
•
•
•
•

How will we know that a change is an improvment? (See Appendix A: Sample measures)
What are our measures?
What is our current performance?
Internal Benchmark (To what internal, e.g., unit-based, JHH-based, measure will we compare our performance?)
External Benchmark (To what external, e.g., outside JHH, measure will we compare our performance?)

What changes can we make that will result in improvement?

The Johns Hopkins Hospital Performance Improvement Workbook

PDSA: PLAN (See Appendix C)

Statement of goals (aim)

Data collection plan
What data needs to be collected?
Who will collect/analyze data?
How/where are data obtained? (e.g., chart review, audit tool, patient interview, data extraction)
When/how often are data obtained?

Identify the current process. (see Appendix B: Flow Charting Tips)

Choose one small change in the current process to pilot test.

PDSA: Plan-DO (See Appendix C)

Document PROBLEMS and UNEXPECTED OBSERVATIONS as we carry out the pilot.

Document OBSERVATIONS as we begin data analysis. (Are the data telling us what we need to know?)

The Johns Hopkins Hospital Performance Improvement Workbook

PDSA: Plan-Do-**STUDY** (See Appendix C)

Complete ANALYSIS of the data. (What have we learned?)

COMPARE the data to our predictions. (Did original outcomes improve?)

PDSA: Plan-Do-Study-**ACT**

If change was successful, how will we BUILD this change into our DAILY WORK ROUTINES?

How will we communicate this change?

If change was not successful, what was the SOURCE OF FAILURE? (See Appendix D)

Choose NEXT CHANGE in the current process to pilot test.

The Johns Hopkins Hospital Performance Improvement Workbook

Appendix A: Sample Measures (Metrics)

This list is NOT all-inclusive. It is intended to give you a general idea of the types of measures included on the JHH Performance profile. When choosing your measures, it is best to choose at least one process measure and one outcome measure.

CLINICAL (clinical effectiveness, patient safety)
Heart failure patients discharged home with written instructions or educational material addressing activity level, diet, discharge medications, follow-up appointment, weight monitoring, and what to do if symptoms worsen. (process measure)
15-day unplanned readmission rate (outcome measure)
Nosocomial infection rate (outcome measure)
Timeliness of antibiotic administration for pneumonia inpatients (process measure)
Inpatient fall-related injury rate (outcome measure)

SERVICE (workplace quality, patient satisfaction)
Overall employee satisfaction rate (outcome measure)
Supply management service score (process measure)
Days lost due to injury per 100 employees (outcome measure)
Overall inpatient satisfaction rate (outcome measure)
Number of patient complaints (outcome measure)

FISCAL (financial performance, revenue recovery)	
Average length of stay (outcome measure)	Collection rate (outcome measure)
Case mix index, hospital total (outcome measure)	Administrative denial rate (outcome measure)
JHH charge/case (outcome measure)	Clinical denial recovery rate (outcome measure)

INFRASTRUCTURE (access)	
Red alert hours (outcome measure)	Cancelled ambulatory procedure rate (outcome measure)
Yellow alert hours (outcome measure)	OR start time compliance rate (outcome measure)
HAL turnaway rate (outcome measure)	Surgical procedures (outcome measure)
Rate of ED walkouts (outcome measure)	ED visits (outcome measure)

The Johns Hopkins Hospital Performance Improvement Workbook

Appendix B: Frequently Used Flow Charting Symbols and Sample Flow Chart

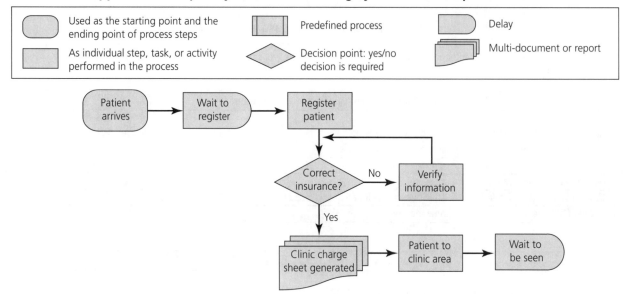

Used as the starting point and the ending point of process steps	Predefined process	Delay
As individual step, task, or activity performed in the process	Decision point: yes/no decision is required	Multi-document or report

Appendix C: Keys to Success

PLAN
- <u>Choosing a project</u>: discuss failures in existing systems with managers (physician, nurse, and administrative).
- <u>Deciding which project to do first</u>: consider the probability of harm from the system failure and the severity of the harm.
- <u>Setting goals</u>:
  1. Make goals explicit.
  2. Include both internal benchmarks (e.g., "reduce the rate of medication errors by 50") and external benchmarks (e.g., have the lowest rate of hospital-acquired pneumonia in the country).
- <u>Benchmarking</u>:
  1. Obtain baseline data and create a run chart.
  2. Run chart template is available on the Hopkins intranet.
- <u>Choosing which change to test</u>:
  1. Identify key steps in the process. These could be processes of care that are evidence-based (e.g., handwashing) or bottlenecks (e.g., obtaining consent before surgery).
  2. Ensure that the key process occurs.
     a) Reduce the number of steps in the process (complexity).
     b) Have separate mechanisms in place to ensure that key processes are done (e.g., if providing flu shots for all caregivers is important, then have department heads <u>and</u> infection control practitioners help ensure that this occurs).
  3. While changes can be large, it is best to test on a small scale. (e.g., we can try the change on one physician's patients, or patients on one unit for one week.)
- <u>Measuring success</u>:
  1. Choose measures to evaluate success of process changes.
  2. Areas of focus at JHH are clinical (effectiveness/patient safety), service (workplace quality/patient satisfaction), fiscal (financial performance/revenue recovery), and infrastructure (access). See Appendix A for sample measures.

DO
- To decide whether data are telling us what we want to know, answer the following questions, as appropriate:
  - Is the process clear (when, what, how)?
  - Are tasks consistently carried out?
  - Is there role confusion?
  - Are resources in place (supplies, equipment, physical environment)?
  - Are work outcomes accurate, error-free, timely?
  - Is feedback communicated in a timely manner to the appropriate individuals?
  - Is process organized, appropriate pace, tasks not interrupted?

STUDY
- Choose the best display of your data to show if the intended result is achieved.

The Johns Hopkins Hospital Performance Improvement Workbook

Appendix D: Failure Source Anaylsis Grid

To determine why the selected changes(s) were not successful, identify causes and determine appropriate solution strategies.

SKILL/KNOWLEDGE DEFICIT	CAUSE	
1. Some People Lack Knowledge or Skill *Solution Strategy:* Train or brief people; Modify hiring selection criteria.	❑ Don't know responsibilities/roles. ❑ Were not qualified to do the job when hired. ❑ Don't know/understand performance expectations. ❑ Don't know importance of their performance to others.	❑ Don't know JHH/department/unit goals. ❑ Don't know how to perform tasks. ❑ Don't know when to perform tasks. ❑ Don't perform tasks often enough to develop proficiency.
2. Inadequate Training *Solution Strategy:* Train people, or give them more practice training.	❑ Training not given to everyone needing it. ❑ Time from training to skill application too long. ❑ Training not performance-based. ❑ Training content doesn't match real job.	❑ Inadequate practice. ❑ Training is unstructured. ❑ No measurement/proof of competency. ❑ Inadequate time spent in formal training.
3. Ineffective Job or Task Aids *Solution Strategy:* Create or improve job aids.	❑ Don't tell when to do steps of task. ❑ Don't tell how to do steps of task. ❑ Not detailed enough. ❑ Not current.	❑ Too long. ❑ Too confusing to use. ❑ People don't have access to job aids. ❑ People don't know job aids exist.

PROCESS DEFICIT	CAUSE	
1. Inappropriate Workload *Solution Strategy:* Revise expectations or staffing standards.	❑ Workload too heavy. ❑ Not enough time to complete tasks. ❑ Performance expectations unclear or non-existent.	❑ Performance expectations too high. ❑ Performance expectations not mutually agreed upon.
2. Needed Elements Not Available *Solution Strategy:* Get resources in place.	❑ Tools, materials, equipment lacking, broken, not current. ❑ Assistance from others lacking.	❑ Data and information missing, late, incomplete, inaccurate. ❑ People don't supply needed product.
3. Inadequate Working Conditions *Solution Strategy:* Improve conditions.	❑ Working conditions hinder work: lighting, temperature, space, noise, safety, cleanliness.	
4. Inefficient Work Design *Solution Strategy:* Customize to identified cause.	❑ Frequent interruptions/competing priorities. ❑ Varies with time of day, day of week. ❑ Insufficient empowerment to do task. ❑ Insufficient time to perform task.	❑ Inadequate opportunity to troubleshoot outcomes. ❑ Inadequate opportunity to correct errors. ❑ Checks & balances in the wrong places. ❑ Critical decisions occur too early/late.

The Johns Hopkins Hospital Performance Improvement Workbook

Appendix D: Failure Source Anaylsis Grid, continued

FEEDBACK AND MOTIVATION	CAUSE	
1. Task in Question, or Some Aspect of it, Is Punitive *Solution Strategy:* Change procedure to remove punishing parts.	❏ Dangerous, unsafe conditions. ❏ Very difficult behavior involved. ❏ Socially negative – peers punish, against culture.	❏ Stressful; high consequences of error. ❏ Task is boring, repetitive. ❏ Discrepancy between known professional standards & JHH culture.
2. Inadequate Performance Feedback *Solution Strategy:* Improve quality and/or timeliness of feedback.	❏ Doesn't occur often enough to reinforce improvement. ❏ Not timely enough to change performance.	❏ Doesn't show differences between expected and actual behavior. ❏ Not balanced (positive and negative feedback).
3. Consequences Do Not Support Desired Performance *Solution Strategy:* Re-balance consequences.	❏ Positive consequence for competing behavior. ❏ Positive consequence for incorrect behavior.	❏ Negative consequence for correct behavior.
4. Task/Role Confusion *Solution Strategy:* Clarify role/task.	❏ Perception that task lacks value. ❏ Doesn't understand task.	❏ Disagrees how task should be done. ❏ Believes someone else should do task.

Index

page numbers followed by f or t denote figures or tables respectively

A

Abstracts, publication of
 editorial review, 76–77
 guidelines for publication, 75–76
 reasons for rejection, 77
 steps in publishing a manuscript, 75
 submitting the abstract, 70–71, 70t
 target a specific journal, 75
Agency for Healthcare Research and Quality
 (AHRQ), 34, 63
Aggressive patient, 107–119
 act
  data collection as a treatment team
   communication tool, 118
  performance improvement data collection
   and analysis, 118
 aggression screening/assessment tool, 109f
 aggressive events, 108, 110
 background, 108
 conclusion, 119
 do
  Phipps Aggression Screening Tool (PAST),
   109f, 113
  Phipps Aggressive Patient Management
   Indicator (PAPMI), 113, 114–115f, 115
  revision of the assessment tool, 113
 example, 107–108
 plan
  Brief Psychiatric Rating Scale (BPRS), 111
  command hallucinations and delusions as
   indicator, 113
  consequences of patient aggression, 110
  consequences of repeated violence, 111
  evaluating potential for violence, 110–113
  MacArthur Violence Risk Assessment
   Study, 112
  Mini Mental State Examination (MMSE),
   111
  Nurses' Observational Scale for Inpatient
   Evaluation (NOSIE), 111
  Overt Aggression Scale (OAS), 111
  percent of patients admitted to JHH with
   history of aggression, 112
  revision of data collection tools, 112
 study
  aggressive events per shift, 116, 116f
  care plan interventions, 116, 116f
  frequency of interventions post-event, 116,
   117f, 118
  PAST and PAMPI completed, 115
AHRQ (Agency for Healthcare Research and
 Quality), 34, 63
Alarm systems, clinical, patient safety goals to
 improve effectiveness of, 19t
American Nurses Association (ANA)
 measuring patient safety, 21
 professional commitment of nurses, 10
 Safety and Quality Initiative, 63

American Society of Anesthesiologists (ASA) score, 57
American Society of PeriAnesthesia Nurses (ASPAN), 78
Analytical skills, competency in, 37
Antimicrobial-resistant microorganisms, and nosocomial infections, 18
Association for periOperative Registered Nurses (AORN), 10

B

Berwick, Donald, 3
Bloodstream infection (BSI), 18
Brief Psychiatric Rating Scale (BPRS), 111
Buerhaus, P., 23

C

Care bundle, 83
Centers for Disease Control (CDC), assessing improvements in hand hygiene adherence, 20
Central-line associated bloodstream infection (BSI), 18
Champion, 32
    physician as, 42
Checklists, use of, 34
    for chemotherapy administration, 97, 98f
Chemotherapy safety, 95–105
    act
        changes being initiated, 103
        chemotherapy survey tool, 103, 105
        Failure Modes Effects Analysis (FEMA), 103, 105
        ongoing review of errors and of the system, 103
        staff education, 105
    background, 96
    chemotherapy process, 96
    do
        attending physician treatment plan, 101
        chemotherapy administration checklist, 97, 98f
        chemotherapy/biotherapy orders, defined, 101
        development of preprinted standard chemotherapy order sets, 99, 100f, 101
        drug-specific parameters, 101, 102f
        easy access to online resources, 102–103
        FEMA chemotherapy process, 105
        handwritten physician chemotherapy orders, a high-risk practice, 99
        hospital-wide education, 97
        near-miss error reporting data, 97, 99
        Oncology Clinical Tools Icon, 103, 104f
        policy review, 97
        requirements for a reference treatment plan, 101
    independent validation of pertinent lab values, 95
    JHH Chemotherapy Policy, revised, 96

plan, 96–97
    root cause analysis and performance improvement initiatives outcome, 96
    study: near-miss errors, 103
City resources for conducting a safety project, 123–124
Clinical performance and public accountability, assessments of, 7
Clinical resources, 124–127
Code of Ethics for Nurses (ANA), 2001, 1–2
Codification of safety principles, 14–15
Collaboration, interdisciplinary, 36–37
    barriers and success strategies, 93t
Command hallucinations and delusions as indicator of potential violence, 113
Communication
    among caregivers, patient safety goals for improving effectiveness of, 19t
    barriers to and success strategies, 93t
    as contributing factor to safety problems, 33
    use of a daily goals and objectives sheet, 34
Complications
    increase cost, 8f
    increase mortality, 8f
Comprehensive Accreditation Manual for Hospitals: The Official Handbook, safety issues, 15
Contributing factors to safety problems, 33t
    suggestions to address frequent contributing factors, 34
Crossing the Quality Chasm: A New Health System for the 21st Century, 2, 35

D

"Daily Goals" form, 84–85
Data analyst, 32
Data collection
    barriers and success strategies, 93t
    cost of *vs.* potential benefit from the improvement, 82
    data analysis plan, 59
    data representing categories, 59
    ethical implications of, 56
    evaluating the feasibility of, 56
    identifying data sources, 57
Data management, competency in, 37
Deaths
    annual preventable deaths in U.S. hospitals, 3
    from hospital-acquired infection, 18
Deep venous thrombosis (DVT), 80
Deming, W. Edwards, 17, 43
Dickerson-Hazard, N., 23
Director of Nursing (DON), internal dissemination of findings, 69
Dissemination of findings, 67–78

comparative study between bedside and laboratory hemoglobin testing, 67, 77–78

external dissemination, 68, 69–77

external opportunities for disseminating results of safety projects, 69

oral presentations, 71t

logistics, 72–73

method, 72

technology, 72

time, 72

poster presentation, 73t

advantages over oral presentations, 74

preparation of the poster, 74

size and media, 74

time allowed, 74

type of display, 73–74

publication

editorial review, 76–77

guidelines for publication, 75–76

reasons for rejection, 77

steps in publishing a manuscript, 75

target a specific journal, 75

submitting the abstract, 70–71, 70t

importance of, 67–68

internal dissemination, 68, 69

mechanisms to disseminate information, 68

objectives of the chapter, 68

DMAIC, 40

Document results and share the stories, 35

DVT (Deep venous thrombosis), 80

E

EBP (evidence-based practice), 4–5, 5t

Education

Oncology Nursing Society's Chemotherapy and Biotherapy Course, 105

professional education and development strategies, 5, 5t

science of safety education, 30–31

Error reduction, concepts of, 9t

Errors. *See* Medical errors; Near-miss errors, chemotherapy safety

Ethical considerations, data collection, 56

Evidence-based practice (EBP), 4–5, 5t

medication-related events, 15

Evolutionary improvement methods, 40

Executive Adopt a Unit program, 32

External resources, networking with, 34

F

Failure Modes Effects Analysis (FEMA), chemotherapy process, 103, 105

Flowcharting, 42–43, 42f

G

Government resources for conducting a safety project, 123–124

H

Hand hygiene, improvements in adherence to, 20

HAPI (Health and Psychosocial Instruments), 60

Head of bed elevation (HOB), 80

Health and Psychosocial Instruments (HAPI), 60

Healthcare-acquired infections, patient safety goals for reducing, 19t

Health Insurance Portability and Accountability Act (HIPPA), patients' rights to privacy, 56

Hemoglobin values, comparative study between bedside and laboratory hemoglobin testing, 67, 77–78

Hospital-acquired infection, 18, 20

rate of per 1000 patient days, 18

Hospitals, annual preventable deaths in U.S. hospitals, 3

I

Identification, patient, safety goals for improving accuracy of, 19t

Independent redundancy, 83, 89

Indexes, resources, 124–127

Institute for Healthcare Improvement (IHI), 34, 80

Institute of Medicine (IOM)

definition of quality, 2

report on medical errors (1999), 9, 31

reports on patient safety, 2

use of information technology, 35

Institute of Safe Medication Practices (ISMP), 15

Institutional Review Board, approval, 56

Instrument

defined, 53t

evaluation, 59t

Intensive care unit (ICU). *See also* Mechanical ventilation; Medication reconciliation in the ICU

preventable adverse events in, 79–80

six steps to select and develop quality measures in the ICU

conducting a systematic literature review, 55

evaluating validity and reliability, 57, 59

pilot measures

selecting, 57

testing, 59–60

selecting specific types of outcomes to evaluate, 55–57

target dates, 55t

writing design specifications for the measures, 56–57, 58t

Internal resources, networking with, 34

Intravenous (IV) infusion pumps

   case study: events involving IV sedation bolus administration

     how would we know change was an improvement

      current process, 47–48

      measures, 48

     PDSA

      act, 49

      do, 48

      plan, 48

      study, 48

     what changes would result in improvement

      proposed changes, 48

      selected change to pilot test, 48

     what were we trying to accomplish?

      aim, 47

      motivation, 47

      team members, 47

   goals to improve safety of, 19t

   medication errors in use of, 39

   "smart-pump" technology, 48–49

ISMP Medication Safety Alert, 15

J

Johns Hopkins Hospital. *See also* Performance improvement (PI); Performance improvement (PI) workbook

   Chemotherapy Policy, revised, 96 (*See also* Chemotherapy safety)

   clinical patient safety performance measures, 22t

Joint Commission of Healthcare Organizations (JCAHO), 34

   cycle for improving performance, 40

   Patient Safety Goals, 18, 19t

   Sentinel Event Alerts, 15

   staffing effectiveness measures, 21

K

Keeping Patients Safe: Transforming the Work Environment for Nurses (2004), 2

L

Likert scale questionnaire, 29, 30t

M

MacArthur Violence Risk Assessment Study, 112

Measure, defined, 53t

Measurement, defined, 53t

Measurement of improvement changes, 42–43

Measuring patient safety, 51–64

   safety measures of structure, process, and outcome, 60–63

     examples of, 61t

     nurse-sensitive outcomes, 63, 63t

     outcome measures, 61–62, 62t

     process measures, 61–62, 62t

     quality measures for organizational use, 63

     risk adjustment, 62

     structure measure for presence of equipment in OR, 61

   selecting a patient safety measure

     choose the measure, 54

     concept definitions, 52, 53t

     establish a set of criteria, 54–55

     identifying the problem to be measured, 53, 54t

     locating examples of measures, 60

     metric or measure defined, 53

     patient safety measure defined, 52

     process of developing a quality measure, 53

     six steps to select and develop quality measures in the ICU

      conducting a systematic literature review, 55

      evaluating validity and reliability, 57, 59

      pilot measures

       selecting, 57

       testing, 59–60

      selecting specific types of outcomes to evaluate, 55–57

      target dates, 55t

      writing design specifications for the measures, 56–57, 58t

     team decisions, 54–60

   using a system approach, and detailing specific aims and measurement, 51–52

Mechanical ventilation, 79–85

   changes that would result in an improvement

     act, 84–85

     bundle care processes, 83

     "Daily Goals" form, 84–85

     do, 84

     independent redundancy, 83

interventions to improve complexity, 82–83

plan, 84

study, 84

team approach, 83

gap between available evidence and best practice, 80

patient outcome results of using all four processes, 80

reaching the goals

choosing measures that reflect changes we could make, 81

choosing what to be measured, 81

data collection, cost of *vs.* potential benefit from the improvement, 82

evaluating outcome measures, 82

evaluating process measures, 82

evidenced-based process measures, 81

randomized clinical trials (RCT), 81

variability in performance, 81

therapies or processes to reduce adverse events, 80

Medical errors. *See also* Near-miss errors, chemotherapy safety

flaws in the system leading to, example, 3–4

IOM report, (1999), 9, 31

ongoing review of errors and of the system, 103

reduction, concepts of, 9t

Medical resources, 124–127

Medication reconciliation in the ICU, 89–94

act, 91–92

background, 89–90

concept of independent redundancy, 89

do, 90

intervention rate over 2 years, 92f

lessons learned, 93, 94t

barriers and success strategies, 92–93, 93t

percentage of patients leaving WICU with potential medication errors, 91f

plan, 90

study, 90–91

Medication-related events, evidence-based source of, 15

Medication safety, 20–21. *See also* Medication reconciliation in the ICU

patient safety goals for using high-alert medications, 19t

Microsoft Visio Professional 2002, 42

Mini Mental State Examination (MMSE), 111

Mission statement, safety, 14, 15

Model for Improvement, 40–47, 41f

N

National Database of Nursing Quality Indicators (NDNQI), 63

National Nosocomial Infections Surveillance System (NNISS), 20

National Quality Measurement and Reporting System, Strategic Framework Board, criteria for evaluating quality measures, 54–55

Near-miss errors, chemotherapy safety

reporting data, 97, 99

study, 103

NNISS (National Nosocomial Infections Surveillance System), 20

NOSIE (Nurses' Observational Scale for Inpatient Evaluation), 111

Nosocomial infections. *See* Hospital-acquired infection

Nurses, role of in planning a safety project, 35–37, 36t

competency in data management and analytical skills, 37

fostering collaboration and patient-centered health care, 36–37

making the vision a reality, 36

Nurse-sensitive outcomes, 63, 63t

Nurses' Observational Scale for Inpatient Evaluation (NOSIE), 111

Nursing directories, resources, 124–127

Nursing-sensitive patient outcomes indicators, 21

O

OAS (Overt Aggression Scale), 111

Occupational Safety and Health Administration (OSHA), work practice guidelines for aggression assessment, 119

Oncology Clinical Tools Icon, 103, 104f

Oncology Nursing Society, Chemotherapy and Biotherapy Course, 105

Online resources, for oncology providers, 102–103

Oral presentations, 71t

logistics, 72–73

method, 72

technology, 72

time, 72

organizational goals for improvement in 2003, 17

"Or the risk thereof," defined, 18

OSHA (Occupational Safety and Health Administration), work practice guidelines for aggression assessment, 119

Outcome measures, 61–62, 62t

evaluating, 82

Outcomes, defined, 53t

Overt Aggression Scale (OAS), 111

P

PACU (Post-anesthesia care unit), comparative study between bedside and laboratory hemoglobin testing, 67, 77–78
PAPMI (Phipps Aggressive Patient Management Indicator), 113, 114–115f, 115
PAST (Phipps Aggression Screening Tool), 109f, 113
Patient-centered care, quality of care, 6
Patient identification, safety goals for improving accuracy of, 19t
Patient safety, and healthcare quality
  chapter objectives, 2
  improving quality of care, 4–9
    evidence-based practice (EBP), 4–5
    patient-centered care, 6
    patient safety as a measure of healthcare quality, 7
      complications increase cost, 8f
      complications increase mortality, 8f
      concepts of error reduction, 8f
    performance improvement by measurement, 6–7
    professional education and development strategies, 5, 5t
    quality improvement model (Nolan), 7
    regular assessments of clinical performance and public accountability, 7
    total quality management (TQM), 6
  nurse's role, 1–2
  quality
    defined, 2
    six domains of, 3
  scope of the problem
    annual preventable deaths in U.S. hospitals, 3
    flaws in the system leading to medical error, example, 3–4
  why nurses should measure safety outcomes, 9–10
Patient Safety Goals (JCAHO), 18, 19t
PDSA. *See* Plan-Do-Study-Act (PDSA) model
Pediatric intensive care unit (PICU), delayed maximizing bronchodilation therapy, 121
Peer review, abstracts, 70
Peptic ulcer (PUD) prophylaxis, 80
Performance improvement (PI)
  alignment of safety and, 15–17
    institution of a staff-centered safety infrastructure, 16
    JHH PI committee structure, 16–17, 16f
  clinical patient safety performance measures, 22t
  codification of safety principles, 14–15
  day-to-day challenges of nurses, 13–14
  developing safer systems, 2
  enabling staff participation, 17
  Ethical Framework for Safety, 14–15

  information that can generate policy change, 15
  priority topics for improvement, 17–21
    hospital-acquired infection, 18, 20
    medication safety, 20–21
    nurse-sensitive safety measures, 21
    sentinel events and patient safety goals, 18
  recommendations for Nurse leaders, 23
  safety mission statement, 14, 15
  to support patient safety, 13–23
  use of a monthly PI Profile, 22
Performance Improvement (PI) workbook, 137–144
  failure source analysis grid, 143–144
  flow charting symbols and sample flow chart, 142
  keys to success, 142
  sample measures (metrics), 141
Phipps Aggression Screening Tool (PAST), 109f, 113
Phipps Aggressive Patient Management Indicator (PAPMI), 113, 114–115f, 115
PICU (Pediatric intensive care unit), delayed maximizing bronchodilation therapy, 121
PI improvement committee structure, 16
Pittsburgh Regional Healthcare Initiative coalition, 32
Plan and implement improvements, 33–35
Plan-Do-Study-Act (PDSA) model, 34, 53
  case study: events involving IV sedation bolus administration, PDSA
    act, 49
    do, 48
    plan, 48
    study, 48
Planning a safety project, 27–37
  assumptions and realities, 28
  a comprehensive patient safety program, 28–35
    eight step process, 29f
    framework for evaluating contributing factors, 31–33, 33t
    step 1: safety climate survey, 29–30, 30t
    step 2: the science of safety education, 30–31
    step 3: staff survey, 31
    step 4: taking an in-depth look, 31–33
    step 5: plan and implement improvements, 33–35
    step 6 & 7: document results and share the stories, 35
    step 8: resurvey staff, 35
  objectives, 28
  role of the nurse, 35–37, 36t
    competency in data management and analytical skills, 37
    fostering collaboration and patient-centered health care, 36–37
    making the vision a reality, 36
Pneumonia. *See also* Mechanical ventilation
  ventilator-associated, 18, 79

Point-of-care testing, for preoperative patients, 67, 68
Post-anesthesia care unit (PACU), comparative study
    between bedside and laboratory hemoglobin
    testing, 67, 77–78
Poster presentations, 73t
  advantages over oral presentations, 74
  preparation of the poster, 74
  size and media, 74
  time allowed, 74
  type of display, 73–74
Process measures, 61–62, 62t
  evaluating, 82
  evidenced-based, 81
Professional education and development strategies, 5, 5t
Professional organizations and associations, resources,
    127–133
Project leader, 32
Project team, support for, roles
  champion, 32
  data analyst, 32
  project leader, 32
Protocols, use of, 34
Publication of abstracts. See Abstracts, publication of
PUD (Peptic ulcer prophylaxis), 80

Q

Quality
  defined, 2
  six domains of, 3
Quality improvement model (Nolan), 7
Quality Indicator Project, 57, 63
Quality measures for organizational use, 63

R

Randomized clinical trials (RCT), 81
Rapid cycle safety improvement
  case study: events involving IV sedation bolus
    administration
    how would we know change was an improvement
      current process, 47–48
      measures, 48
    PDSA
      act, 49
      do, 48
      plan, 48
      study, 48
    what changes would result in improvement
      proposed changes, 48
      selected change to pilot test, 48
    what were we trying to accomplish?
      aim, 47
      motivation, 47
      team members, 47
  current quality improvement methods, 40
    Model for Improvement, 40–47, 41f
      contributors to unsuccessful change, 47t, 46
      PDSA approach, 43–47, 44t
        act, 46
        do, 45, 45t
        plan, 44
        study, 45–46
      questions
        how will we know that change is an
          improvement, 42–43
        what are we trying to accomplish, 41–42
        what changes will result in improvement, 43
  evolutionary methods, 40
  objectives of the chapter, 39–40
  revolutionary methods, 40
Re-engineering, 40
Research resources, 133–134
Resistance to change, barriers and success strategies, 93t
Resources for conducting a safety project
  city, state, and federal government, 123–124
  external sources, 122
  internal sources, 122
  medical and nursing directories, indexes, and clinical
    resources, 124–127
  miscellaneous safety sites, 134–136
  professional organizations and associations, 127–133
  research, 133–134
  safety resources, 122
  search engines, 136
Revolutionary improvement methods, 40
Risk adjustment, 62

S

Safety, defined, 53t
Safety and Quality Initiative (ANA), 21, 63
Safety Attitudes Questionnaire, 29–30
Safety climate survey, 29–30, 30t
Safety measures of structure, process, and outcome,
    60–63
  examples of, 61t
  nurse-sensitive outcomes, 63, 63t
  outcome measures, 61–62, 62t
  process measures, 61–62, 62t
  quality measures for organizational use, 63
  risk adjustment, 62
  structure measure for presence of equipment in OR, 61
Safety mission statement, 14, 15

Safety sites, resources for conducting a safety project, 134–136
Science of safety education, 30–31
Search engines, resources for conducting a safety project, 136
Sentinel events
 defined, 18
 and patient safety goals, 18, 19t
 Sentinel Event Advisory Group, 18
 Sentinel Event Alerts, 15
Serious injury, defined, 18
Shewhart, W.A., 43
Sidney Kimmel Comprehensive Cancer Center (SKCCC), 96
 development of preprinted standard chemotherapy order sets, 99, 100f, 101
Six Sigma, 40
"Smart-pump" technology, 48–49
Staff surveys, 31, 35
State resources for conducting a safety project, 123–124
Structure measure for presence of equipment in OR, 61
Surgical site infection, 18
System and processes of care, in-depth look at, 31–33

T

Team approach, 83
Technological supports, 35
Time, barriers and success strategies, 93t
To Err is Human: Building a Better Health Care System, 2, 31
Total quality management (TQM), 6

U

Urinary catheter-associated urinary tract infection (UTI), 18

V

Variability in performance, 81
Ventilation. *See* Mechanical ventilation
"Ventilator bundle," 84
Vice President of Patient Care Services (VP), internal dissemination of findings, 69
Violence, patient. *See* Aggressive patient

W

Weinberg Intensive Care Unit (ICU). *See* Medication reconciliation in the ICU
Workbook, Performance Improvement. *See* Performance Improvement (PI) workbook
Working conditions, optimizing, 34
Wrong site, wrong patient, wrong procedure surgery, patient safety goals to eliminate, 19t